S0-CVL-701

Springer Series in Optical Sciences Volume 34

Edited by Koichi Shimoda

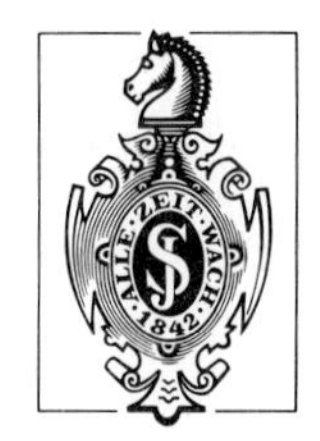

Springer Series in Optical Sciences

1 **Solid-State Laser Engineering**
By. W. Koechner

2 **Table of Laser Lines in Gases and Vapors**
3rd Edition
By R. Beck, W. Englisch, and K. Gürs

3 **Tunable Lasers and Applications**
Editors: A. Mooradian, T. Jaeger, and P. Stokseth

4 **Nonlinear Laser Spectroscopy**
By V. S. Letokhov and V. P. Chebotayev

5 **Optics and Lasers**
An Engineering Physics Approach
By M. Young

6 **Photoelectron Statistics**
With Applications to Spectroscopy and Optical Communication
By B. Saleh

7 **Laser Spectroscopy III**
Editors: J. L. Hall and J. L. Carlsten

8 **Frontiers in Visual Science**
Editors: S. J. Cool and E. J. Smith III

9 **High-Power Lasers and Applications**
2nd Printing
Editors: K.-L. Kompa and H. Walther

10 **Detection of Optical and Infrared Radiation**
2nd Printing
By R. H. Kingston

11 **Matrix Theory of Photoelasticity**
By P. S. Theocaris and E. E. Gdoutos

12 **The Monte Carlo Method in Atmospheric Optics**
By G. I. Marchuk, G. A. Mikhailov, M. A. Nazaraliev, R. A. Darbinian, B. A. Kargin, and B. S. Elepov

13 **Physiological Optics**
By Y. Le Grand and S. G. El Hage

14 **Laser Crystals** Physics and Properties
By A. A. Kaminskii

15 **X-Ray Spectroscopy**
By B. K. Agarwal

16 **Holographic Interferometry**
From the Scope of Deformation Analysis of Opaque Bodies
By W. Schumann and M. Dubas

17 **Nonlinear Optics of Free Atoms and Molecules**
By D. C. Hanna, M. A. Yuratich, D. Cotter

18 **Holography in Medicine and Biology**
Editor: G. von Bally

19 **Color Theory and Its Application in Art and Design**
By G. A. Agoston

20 **Interferometry by Holography**
By Yu. I. Ostrovsky, M. M. Butusov, G. V. Ostrovskaya

21 **Laser Spectroscopy IV**
Editors: H. Walther, K. W. Rothe

22 **Lasers in Photomedicine and Photobiology**
Editors: R. Pratesi and C. A. Sacchi

23 **Vertebrate Photoreceptor Optics**
Editors: J. M. Enoch and F. L. Tobey, Jr.

24 **Optical Fiber Systems and Their Components**
An Introduction
By A. B. Sharma, S. J. Halme, and M. M. Butusov

25 **High Peak Power Nd : Glass Laser Systems**
By D. C. Brown

26 **Lasers and Applications**
Editors: W. O. N. Guimaraes, C. T. Lin, and A. Mooradian

27 **Color Measurement** Theme and Variations
By D. L. MacAdam

28 **Modular Optical Design**
By O. N. Stavroudis

29 **Inverse Problems of Lidar Sensing of the Atmosphere** By V. E. Zuev and I. E. Naats

30 **Laser Spectroscopy V**
Editors: A. R. W. McKellar, T. Oka, and B. P. Stoicheff

31 **Optics in Biomedical Sciences**
Editors: G. von Bally and P. Greguss

32 **Fiber-Optic Rotation Sensors** and Related Technologies
Editors: S. Ezekiel and H. J. Arditty

33 **Integrated Optics: Theory and Technology**
By R.G. Hunsperger

34 **The High-Power Iodine Laser**
By G. Brederlow, E. Fill, and K. J. Witte

35 **Engineering Optics** By K. Iizuka

36 **Transmission Electron Microscopy**
By L. Reimer

37 **Opto-Acoustic Molecular Spectroscopy**
By V.S. Letokhov and V.P. Zharov

38 **Photon Correlation Techniques**
Editor: E.O. Schulz-DuBois

39 **Optical and Laser Remote Sensing**
By D. K. Killinger and A. Mooradian

G. Brederlow E. Fill K.J. Witte

The High-Power Iodine Laser

With 46 Figures

Springer-Verlag Berlin Heidelberg New York 1983

Dr. GÜNTER BREDERLOW
Dr. ERNST FILL
Dr. KLAUS J. WITTE

Max-Planck-Institut für Quantenoptik,
D-8046 Garching bei München, Fed. Rep. of Germany

ISBN 3-540-11792-X Springer-Verlag Berlin Heidelberg New York
ISBN 0-387-11792-X Springer-Verlag New York Heidelberg Berlin

Offset printing: Beltz Offsetdruck, 6944 Hemsbach/Bergstr. Bookbinding: J. Schäffer OHG, 6718 Grünstadt.
2153/3130-543210

Preface

There have been two major review articles on the iodine laser in the last seven years, "The Photochemical Iodine Laser" by K. Hohla and K. Kompa (*Handbook of Chemical Lasers*, edited by R. Gross and J. Bott, Wiley, New York, 1976) and a SANDIA report (No. 78-1071, 1978) entitled "The Atomic Iodine Laser". Since then, a large body of new material has been published, and practical experience has been gained with large iodine laser systems in Garching (ASTERIX III) and in the USSR. These lasers have now become very reliable tools, especially in fusion-oriented plasma experiments, which represent their main field of application. They can deliver powers in excess of many terawatts per beam and are thus also suited for use in other areas such as X-ray lasers, incoherent X-ray sources, compression of matter and its behaviour at very high densities.

The physics of the iodine laser is now rather well understood, and its technology has reached a standard adequate for the construction of large-scale systems in the multi-hundred kJ range. In view of this new situation, we thought it useful to document the present state of the art in a book. Its contents and the literature cited therein have been chosen to cover those areas which are of main concern in the design and operation of pulsed high-power iodine lasers. These include systems capable of delivering pulses with durations extending from approximately one hundred picoseconds to several nanoseconds. Frequency conversion (2ω, 3ω, 4ω) is also treated. Our book is thus somewhat different from Brown's monograph, *High-Peak-Power Nd: Glass Laser Systems* (Springer Series in Optical Sciences, Vol. 25), in which more emphasis is placed on lasers generating pulses in the range from 30 to 100 ps.

The authors trust that the present book, which contains all the knowledge relevant to high-power iodine lasers accumulated so far, will be useful to many colleagues working in laser fusion or related fields.

Garching, December 1982 *G. Brederlow · E. Fill · K.J. Witte*

Acknowledgements

The authors would like to express particular thanks to Dr. S. Witkowski, Director of the Laser Plasma Division of the Max-Planck-Institut für Quantenoptik (MPQ), for his unfaltering encouragement of this work. They are also grateful to the Board of Directors of the MPQ, Prof. K. Kompa, Prof. H. Walther, and Dr. S. Witkowski for their continued support during the writing of the manuscript.

The assistance of Dr. K. Hohla and Dr. R. Volk in writing the first drafts of those sections indicated in the Table of Contents is gratefully acknowledged. The authors would also like to thank Dr. G. Linford for valuable technical discussions on specialized topics in high-power optics and frequency conversion.

The authors are very grateful to Frau Böckmann for her tireless and painstaking efforts to assure accurate and rapid typing of the manuscript, and to Fräulein Pfister for her excellent execution of the technical drawings. The typing assistance of Frau Hecht and Fräulein Wahl is also gratefully acknowledged.

The authors appreciate the editorial comments made by Dr. G. Linford and Mr. Nicol, and they would also like to thank Dr. Lotsch and Herr Michels of Springer-Verlag for their cooperation and skillful assistance in editing the manuscript.

The appreciation of the authors also goes to the Asterix team: H. Baumhacker, E. Gerck, Dr. R. Volk, H. Krause, F. Denk, A. Herrle, G. Keller, H. Stehbeck, M. Grote, and K. Bauer. Without their assistance, this book would not have been possible.

Contents

The sections indicated by an asterisk were written in collaboration with K. Hohla (now Lambda Physik, Göttingen) and R. Volk (Max-Planck-Institut für Quantenoptik, Garching)

1. Introduction

The iodine photodissociation laser was discovered by KASPER and PIMENTEL in 1964 [1.1]. They observed laser action at 1.315 μm during UV flash photolysis of either gaseous CF_3I or CH_3I. In agreement with the results of PORRET and GOODEVE, who in 1938 had already demonstrated that photolysis of CH_3I produces predominantly excited I $(^2P_{1/2})$ atoms [1.2], they interpreted the stimulated emission signals as being due to the $^2P_{1/2} \rightarrow {}^2P_{3/2}$ transition of atomic iodine.

In 1965 the studies of this laser were extended to several other alkyl iodides [1.3]. The most intense emission was found with fluorinated compounds. Some hydrated compounds also exhibited laser action, but at a lower intensity. The high power iodine photodissociation laser is therefore exclusively based on perfluoroalkyl iodides acting as a laser medium.

In an initial theoretical model POLLACK tried to represent the output of an iodine laser as a function of the laser medium pressure [1.4]. It then took quite some time, however, to explain the whole complexity of the processes occurring in an iodine laser. Of major interest were questions about the radiation lifetimes of the excited iodine atoms and the inversion decay process due to collisional quenching. In 1966 many of the collisional deactivation rate constants were already evaluated [1.5]. These measurements were then further extended and refined in the following years.

In 1968 the first studies dealing mainly with the chemical kinetics of the iodine laser were published. These investigations were primarily concerned with the effect of the chemical and photochemical processes on the inversion density. They also dealt with the processes involved in the self--regeneration of the laser medium and with the determination of the conditions under which decomposition of the laser medium is caused by the pumping process. It has since been possible to clarify most of the processes that are important for understanding laser operation.

The actual technical development of the iodine laser and its applications came relatively late. DEMARIA and ULTEE produced laser pulses with energies of up to 60 J in the oscillator mode as early as 1966 [1.6], and pulses in the nanosecond range were obtained in 1968 by FERRAR in a Q-switching and mode-locking experiment [1.7], but the conditions for constructing a high-power laser, which had to be based on the energy storage principle, were still not given.

Although the lifetime of the upper level (which is controlled by collisional deactivation processes) is long enough for energy storage in amplifiers, a sufficiently large amount of inversion energy could not be stored because of the occurrence of parasitic oscillations. Reduction of the gain and hence of the stimulated emission cross-section of the iodine atoms was thus necessary. This was first done by broadening the laser transition using the Zeeman effect [1.8,9]. Later, however, pressure broadening by a buffer gas turned out to be a better method [1.10-12].

Because the extraction efficiency of the stored optical energy strongly depends on the spectrum of the laser pulse, the features resulting from the hyperfine splitting of both levels of the laser transition have also been investigated by numerous authors [1.12-16].

Starting in 1970, a systematic study of the high-power potential of the iodine laser was conducted by HOHLA and KOMPA [1.17]. Somewhat later similar studies were also begun, particularly by BASOV and co-workers [1.18]. These investigations soon revealed that this laser should be well suited to high-power operation and, furthermore, should meet the requirements imposed on high-power lasers for thermonuclear fusion research. The iodine laser possesses features and qualities common to the other two lasers already employed in the laser fusion field, the Nd glass laser and the CO_2 laser. As a gas laser it has some of the important properties of the CO_2 laser, and because of its wavelength and pump technology it is also similar to the Nd glass laser. The advanced level of development of these two laser systems therefore made it then possible to benefit from the available technologies, thus allowing rapid development of the iodine laser.

By 1976 the feasibility of the iodine laser for high-power operation had already been demonstrated in several laboratories [1.19-23]. In 1978 this laser found its first practical application for fusion-oriented plasma experiments in the single-beam ASTERIX III laser at the Max-Planck-Institut für Quantenoptik (MPQ), Garching [1.24]. These experiments clearly demonstrated that the iodine laser is capable of delivering subnanosecond pulses with multikilojoule energies in a single beam with nearly diffraction-limited beam quality and a high repetition rate, thus showing that this laser is very well suited for laser fusion research.

Apart from this application, the iodine laser is also employed in other fields. For instance, it is used for investigations in chemical kinetics, yielding the fastest method for measuring relaxation times of chemical reactions in aqueous solutions (temperature jump method) [1.25]. Furthermore, other applications also seem feasible since CW operation of the iodine laser has been demonstrated with both UV pumping [1.26,27] and chemical pumping [1.28].

One question of special interest is whether an iodine laser system can be built that will satisfy the requirements of a future laser fusion plant. The chances of realizing such a laser system strongly depend on the attainment of a sufficiently high value of the overall system efficiency and on some technical aspects. Present iodine laser systems have too low an overall efficiency. Here, mainly the efficiencies of the pumping process and of the regeneration process of the laser medium set limitations. There is, however, still a potential for increasing these efficiencies.

Discussion of this topic and of the technical aspects requires knowledge about the basics of the iodine laser. It therefore must be postponed to the end of this monograph. First a survey of the basic features of the iodine laser is given, special emphasis being given to the results of investigations necessary for developing and constructing a high-power iodine laser. In addition, the technical aspects of such a laser are illustrated by describing the layout and the performance of the ASTERIX III system. Since the potential for further improvement as well as the scalability to larger apertures are of great interest in choosing the next generation of fusion lasers, these topics are also described. The discussion then proceeds to the question of whether an iodine laser irradiation system can be realized for a laser fusion power plant.

2. Basic Features

This chapter deals with the physical and chemical prerequisites necessary for understanding the iodine laser.

The first part is concerned with the spectroscopy of the iodine laser transition. The spectroscopic properties of the iodine atom determine the main features of the iodine laser such as wavelength, gain, and bandwidth of the radiation. Spectroscopic aspects also decisively influence the energy extraction and pulse propagation in iodine laser amplifiers.

The second part is devoted to various methods of generating inversion. Technological aspects are considered, e.g. design and performance of xenon flashlamps. Besides the usual pumping method of photodissociating an iodide, some less common methods are also reviewed, such as chemical pumping or gas discharges. These methods are interesting with regard to future development of the iodine laser.

In the last section the usual method of generating inversion, i.e. photodissociation is reviewed in detail. Relevant properties of various iodides will be discussed, the most important feature being the quantum yield for excited iodine production. Chemical reactions following the primary process of photodissociation are then reviewed. The relevance of these reactions to single-shot performance and to the reversibility of the iodine laser cycle will be discussed. Aspects of reversible operation will be treated. The section includes a complete list of reactions and reaction constants necessary for a detailed understanding of iodine laser kinetics.

2.1 Spectroscopy of the Iodine Atom

The iodine atom in its ground state has an electron configuration $5s^2 5p^5$. The p shell is only partially filled, one electron being missing from the rare-gas configuration. In the LS coupling approximation the p shell has an orbital angular momentum quantum number $L = 1$ and a spin quantum number $S = 1/2$. These two angular momenta can combine either parallel or antiparallel, thus forming a fine structure doublet. The total quantum numbers for the two levels of the doublet are $J = 3/2$ for the lower and $J = 1/2$ for the upper level. The shorthand spectroscopic designation for the two states is $^2P_{1/2}$ and $^2P_{3/2}$. The iodine laser transition is the magnetic dipole transition between these two states and can be written as

$$^2P_{1/2} \rightarrow {}^2P_{3/2} \qquad \lambda = 1.3152\ \mu m\ .$$

The transition is electric dipole forbidden since the parity of both states is odd. Because of the low transition probability of the magnetic dipole transition the upper level $^2P_{1/2}$ is metastable, allowing large amounts of energy to be stored in atoms excited to the $^2P_{1/2}$ level.

2.1.1 Spontaneous Emission Lifetime

Employing the one-electron approximation GARSTANG [2.1] obtained an Einstein A coefficient of 7.91 s^{-1} with confidence limits of $\pm$ 20%. When the small quadrupole contribution is included a value of 7.96 s^{-1} is obtained. With allowance for all electrons in the $5p^5$ configuration O'BRIEN and BOWEN [2.2] arrived at an estimate of 9.1 s^{-1} for A which is within the confidence limits proposed by GARSTANG.

The measured A coefficients in older work deviate considerably from these values [2.3] mainly because of quenching by impurities. More recent investigations, however, seem to confirm the theoretical value fairly well. ZUEV et al. [2.4] obtained an A of $5.4 \pm 2\ s^{-1}$. More recently, a value of $A = 9.3\ s^{-1}$ was measured by COMES and PIONTECK [2.5] and a value of $A = 7.7 \pm 0.4\ s^{-1}$ by GALANTI et al. [2.6].

The dependence of the Einstein A coefficient on the buffer gas pressure was investigated by ERSHOV and ZALESSKII [2.7]. They found that the intensity of spontaneous emission from excited iodine atoms increased considerably when a buffer gas such as Xe, Ar or SF_6 was added. This finding was interpreted as a collision-induced radiative transition resulting in an increase of the Einstein A coefficient for the transition $^2P_{1/2} \rightarrow {}^2P_{3/2}$ with increasing buffer gas pressure.

This result, however, was contradicted by GALANTI et al. [2.6], who measured the gain and the linewidth of an amplifier at various pressures of the buffer gases Ar, Xe, and SF_6. It was found that the Einstein A coefficient remained constant at least up to pressures of 4 bar.

The apparent contradiction was resolved in a paper by GERCK and FILL [2.8]. They showed that the enhanced fluorescence was due to an I*-M excimer which is formed in a three-body collision with buffer gas M. The number density of this excimer is extremely low under normal pressure conditions. However, its large transition probability of $\cong 10^7\ s^{-1}$ results in an apparent increase of the fluorescence signal. Because of its low concentration the influence of this excimer on iodine laser kinetics is negligible; it can, however, have an influence on the interpretation of data obtained from fluorescence measurements.

2.1.2 Hyperfine Structure

The iodine laser transition shows hyperfine splitting into 6 lines, as seen in Fig. 2.1. This splitting has important consequences affecting the performance of the iodine laser, as will be discussed later (Sect. 3.3).

The hyperfine spectrum is entirely due to the magnetic moment of the nucleus since the only stable isotope of iodine is ^{127}I. The nuclear spin quantum number of ^{127}I is $I = 5/2$. Different possible orientations of the nuclear angular momentum with respect to the orbital angular momentum result in total angular momentum quantum numbers

$$F = I + J,\ I + J - 1, \dots,\ I - J\ . \qquad (2.1)$$

For the upper level with $J = 1/2$ we therefore obtain splitting into two hyperfine sublevels, whereas the lower laser level with $J = 3/2$ is split into 4 hyperfine sublevels. A selection rule $\Delta F = 0, \pm 1$ applies, resulting in the 6-line spectrum shown in Fig. 2.1. The 6 lines are divided into two groups of 3 lines. Each group originates from a different upper level.

The fluorescence spectrum of the iodine laser transition has been determined by several authors [2.4,9-11]. There are slight differences in some details of the spectrum which have, however, a negligible effect on what is dealt with in the following. The hyperfine structure of the iodine atom as described below uses thus only the data of one of the cited papers, the investigation by ZUEV et al. [2.4].

The main results are contained in Fig. 2.1, which shows the theoretical level spacing and the theoretical and experimental positions of the lines. The splitting constants of the ground state which were obtained experimentally have the values $A_{3/2} = 0.0276\ cm^{-1}$ and $B_{3/2} = 0.000048\ cm^{-1}$.

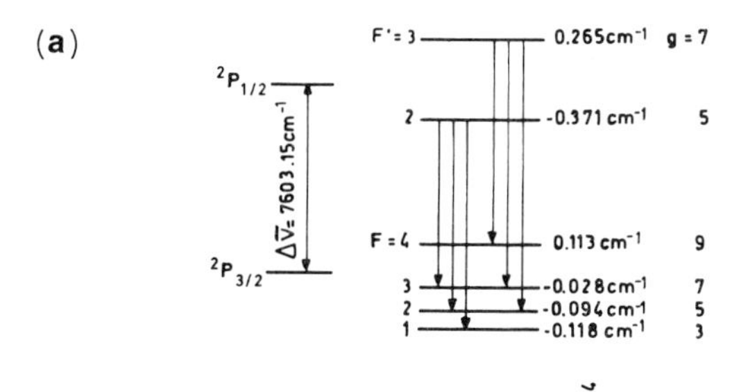

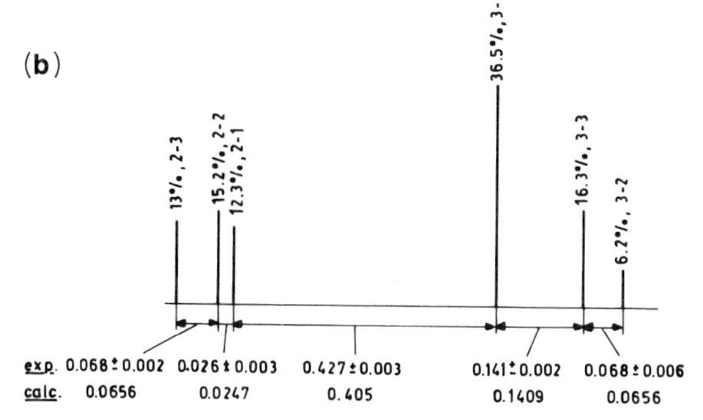

Fig. 2.1a,b. Hyperfine spectrum of the iodine laser transition. (a) Calculated level spacing [2.4]. (b) Comparison of experimental and calculated line positions [2.4]. The relative intensities of the various transitions are theoretically determined [2.4].

The constant $A_{1/2}$ of the excited state was calculated from the fine splitting of the $5p^5\ ^2P$ term of the iodine atom with allowance for the relativistic corrections whereby a value of 0.212 cm^{-1} was obtained. $B_{1/2}$ is zero. With A and B the level splitting ΔE can be determined according to the expression $\Delta E=(1/2)AC+BC(C+1)+\delta$ where $C=F(F+1)-J(J+1)-I(I+1)$ and $\delta=(4/3)BI(I+1)J(J+1)$.

The Einstein A coefficients for the different lines can also be calculated. In the LS coupling approximation the following values are obtained [2.4,12]:

transition F' → F	3-4	3-3	3-2	2-3	2-2	2-1
Einstein A [s^{-1}]	5.1	2.2	0.6	2.4	3.1	2.4
	Σ = 7.9					

The strongest line in the spectrum is the line originating from the upper sublevel with F' = 3 to the lower sublevel with F = 4. This line is usually called the 3-4 line and is ordinarily emitted by an iodine laser oscillator. It is obvious that the hyperfine structure of the iodine spectrum has important consequences for energy extraction and pulse propagation in iodine laser amplifiers. These points will be discussed in Sect. 3.3 on pulse propagation.

2.1.3 Line Broadening and Line Shifts

The actual shape of the iodine spectrum is determined by line broadening and partial overlapping of the individual lines. At low pressures of the iodide and buffer gases (up to about 30 mbar, depending on the gas) the spectrum is Doppler broadened. This broadening, caused by thermal motion of the atoms and independent of pressure, is given by

$$\Delta\nu_D = (2/\lambda)(2\ R\ T\ \ln 2/M)^{1/2}\quad [\mathrm{Hz}] \tag{2.2}$$

where $\Delta\nu_D$ is the full linewidth at half intensity, λ is the wavelength of the iodine laser, T is the temperature of the gas in K, M is the molecular weight of the radiating particle equal to 127 kg/kmol for atomic iodine, and R is the universal gas constant equal to 8314 J/kmol K.

In the Doppler broadened region the shape of an individual line is given by a Gaussian profile.

At room-temperature Doppler broadening of the iodine laser transition amounts to 250 MHz. In a laser the temperature rise due to excitation may increase this Doppler width by a factor of 1.5 to 1.7.

The morc important broadening mechanism under usual laser conditions is pressure broadening. This type of broadening is caused by random-phase changes of the radiating dipoles because of collisions with particles of the iodide and buffer gases.

The shape of a pressure-broadened line is given by a Lorentzian profile. At pressures of up to 4 bar the full width at half maximum (FWHM) $\Delta\nu_p$ of a line broadened by a mixture of different gases can be expressed as

$$\Delta\nu_p = \sum \alpha_i p_i \tag{2.3}$$

where α_i is the pressure broadening coefficient of gas i, and p_i is the partial pressure of gas i.

Pressure broadening is dominant at $\Delta\nu_p \geqq 3\ \Delta\nu_D$. The transition region from Doppler to pressure broadening, where the shape of the line is given by a Voigt profile, is virtually unimportant for laser operation.

The pressure broadening coefficients α_i can be found experimentally using two methods. $\Delta\upsilon_p$ and thus α_i are either directly determined from spectrally resolved measurements of the luminescence or indirectly from gain measurements (Sect. 2.1.4).

Pressure broadening by elastic collisions produces a line shift $\delta\nu_p$ moving the whole spectrum, i.e. all six lines, by the same amount towards shorter wavelengths. Compared to the medium linewidth $\Delta\nu_p$ of single transitions the shift $\delta\nu_p$ is weak; the theoretical prediction of the ratio $\delta\nu_p/\Delta\nu_p$ is $\leqq 0.1$ [2.13]. Experimentally observed values of $\delta\nu_p/\Delta\nu_p$ have been published for n-C_3F_7I [2.14] and the noble gases Ne, Ar and Xe [2.15]. They are also $\leqq 0.1$. Unless a high-pressure oscillator ($\Delta\nu_p \sim 25$ GHz) is coupled to a low-pressure amplifier ($\Delta\nu_p \sim 5$ GHz), the shift $\delta\nu_p$ is of little practical importance.

2.1.4 Stimulated Emission Cross-Section

A stimulated emission cross-section σ_{ij} connecting two levels labelled i (upper) and j (lower) can be defined if the bandwidth of the radiation interacting with the atom is narrow compared with the width of the line. The small-signal gain factor A_{ss} for such radiation is then given by

$$A_{ss} = \exp(\sigma_{ij}\Delta N_{ij}\ell) \tag{2.4}$$

where ℓ is the gain length, and ΔN_{ij} the inversion per cm^3 of the ij transition.

The stimulated emission cross-section at any position within the line is given by

$$\sigma_{ij}(\nu) = (\lambda^2/8\pi)A_{ij}g(\nu) \tag{2.5}$$

where

$$g(\nu) = 2/\{\pi\Delta\nu[1 + 4\,((\nu - \nu_{ij})/\Delta\nu)^2]\} \tag{2.6}$$

is the normalized line-shape function for a pressure-broadened line such that $\int_{-\infty}^{+\infty} g(\nu)\,d\nu = 1$ holds; ν_{ij} is the centre frequency of the ij transition, $\Delta\nu$ the full linewidth at half maximum and ν the carrier frequency of the pulse. The peak value of the induced emission cross-section is obtained at line centre $\nu = \nu_{ij}$ and given by

$$\sigma_{ij} = \lambda^2 A_{ij}/(4\pi^2\Delta\nu)\ . \tag{2.7}$$

In the case of the iodine laser the spectrum consists of six overlapping lines. It is then convenient to introduce an overall cross-section

σ_{tot} defined by [2.16]

$$\sigma_{tot} = 3 \sum \sigma_{ij}(\nu)\Delta N_{ij}/\sum \Delta N_{ij} \tag{2.8a}$$

where the summation is over all six transitions. If it is assumed that all the hyperfine levels are populated by photolysis according to their statistical weights the expression for σ_{tot} can be simplified leading to

$$\sigma_{tot} = A_{tot}\,\lambda^2 G(\nu,\Delta\nu)/(4\pi^2\Delta\nu) \tag{2.8b}$$

where A_{tot} is the *total* transition rate with a theoretical value somewhere between 7.9 and 9.1 s^{-1}. $G(\nu,\Delta\nu)$ is the generalized line-shape function given by (homogeneously broadened line)

$$G(\nu,\Delta\nu) = \frac{5}{12}\sum_{i=1}^{3}\frac{A_{2i}}{A_{tot}}\frac{1}{1+[(\nu-\nu_{2i})/\Delta\nu]^2} + \frac{7}{12}\sum_{i=2}^{4}\frac{A_{3i}}{A_{tot}}\frac{1}{1+[(\nu-\nu_{3i})/\Delta\nu]^2} \quad . \tag{2.8c}$$

In Fig. 2.2 σ_{ij} and σ_{tot} are plotted as a function of ν for three different values of $\Delta\nu$ ($A_{tot} = 8\ s^{-1}$ assumed). For values of $\Delta\nu \leqq 5$ GHz the maximum of σ_{tot} is close to the position of the 3-4 line (see Fig. 3.3). σ_{tot}^{max} decreases more slowly with increasing $\Delta\nu$ than σ_{max} of a single line because of increasing overlap of the lines. In the limit of small linewidths one obtains for $\nu = \nu_{34}$

$$\sigma_{tot}^{max}(\Delta\nu \rightarrow 0) = (7/12)\lambda^2 A_{34}/(4\pi^2\Delta\nu), \tag{2.9}$$

whereas in the limit of large linewidths,

$$\sigma_{tot}^{max}(\Delta\nu \rightarrow \infty) = \lambda^2 A_{tot}/(4\pi^2\Delta\nu) \tag{2.10}$$

holds. Figure 2.3 shows the dependence of σ_{tot} at $\nu = \nu_{34}$ on the buffer gas pressure for a mixture of 100 mbar $i\text{-}C_3F_7I$ and various buffer gases [2.6].

As already mentioned in the previous section, the pressure broadening coefficients α_i can be derived from measurements of σ_{tot} via (2.3,8). Values of α_i for various buffer gases thus obtained ($A_{tot} = 8\ s^{-1}$) are listed in Table 2.1 in which α values based on other measuring tech-

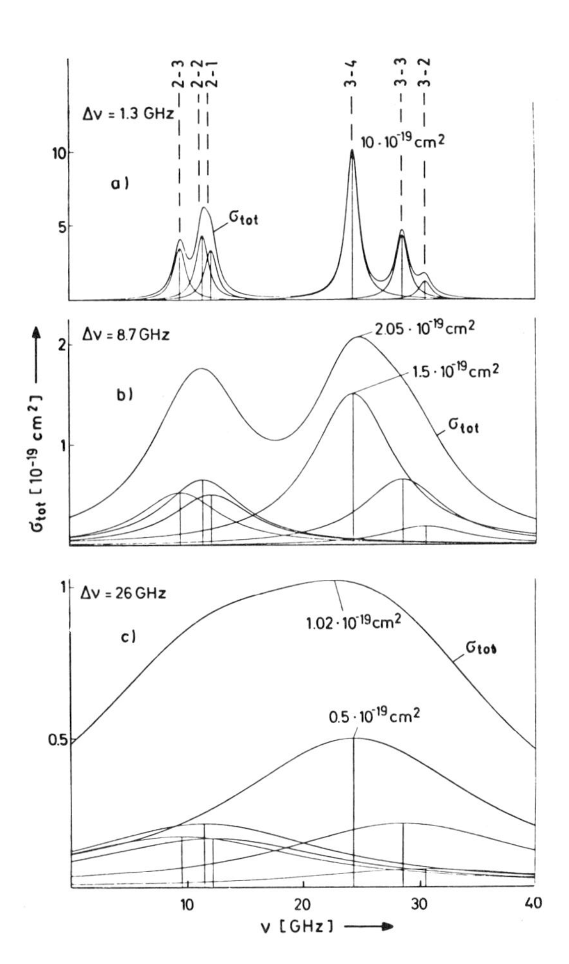

Fig. 2.2. Pressure-broadened iodine laser spectrum

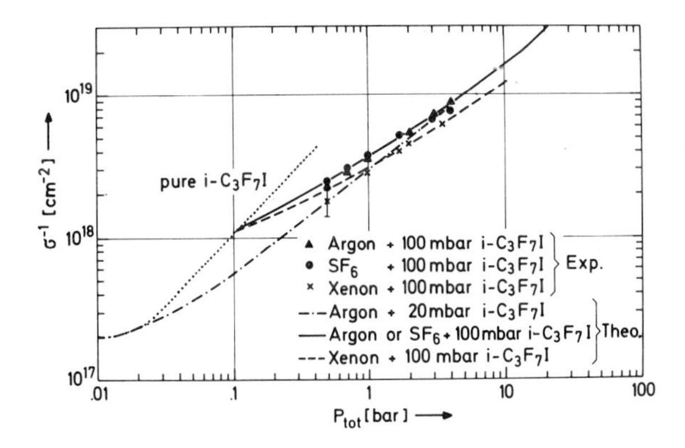

Fig. 2.3. Experimental and calculated values of the stimulated emission cross-section vs buffer gas pressure. The various lines are computed with a value of $A_{tot} = 8\ s^{-1}$ and the following broadening coefficients: 3.8 GHz/bar for Ar and SF_6; 2.5 GHz/bar for Xe; 15 GHz/bar for i-C_3F_7I

Table 2.1. Pressure broadening coefficients of various gases

Gas	α [GHz/bar]	Ref	Gas	α [GHz/bar]	Ref
He	3.1	2.15	SF_6	3.6 - 3.8	2.6
	3.0	2.17		4.9	2.16
Ne	4.5	2.15		4.6	2.20
Ar	4.0	2.4	CO_2	7.7	2.15
	3.8 - 4.2	2.6		7.0	2.16
	3.4	2.14		7.4	2.20
	5.4	2.15	CF_3I	8.5	2.16
	3.6	2.16		7.3	2.21
	3.8	2.18		6.2	2.19
	2.8	2.19		9.0	2.20
	4.6	2.20	$n\text{-}C_3F_7I$	14	2.4
Xe	2.5 - 2.7	2.6		7.8	2.19
	3.0	2.15		18	2.22
	3.2	2.19	$i\text{-}C_3F_7I$	15	2.16
	2.9	2.20		7	2.19
N_2	6.4	2.15	I,I*	12	2.16
	5.0	2.16		(Theoretical estimate)	

Comment pertaining to the measurement methods employed in the references cited:

[2.4] Direct determination of $\Delta\nu$ by luminescence measurements.

[2.6] Direct and independent determination of $\Delta\nu$ and σ_{tot} by A_{ss} and A_{LS} measurements with pulses of variable carrier frequency.

[2.14] α derived from the pressure dependance of the carrier frequency shift of a pulse emitted by a free running oscillator

[2.15] Relative determination of σ_{tot} by A_{ss} measurements with a reference value of $\sigma_{tot}=5\times10^{-18}$ cm^2 for 27 mbar CF_3I. $\Delta\nu$ and thus α were calculated with $A_{tot}=5.5$ s^{-1}. The α values quoted in Table 2.1 are based on $A_{tot}=8$ s^{-1}.

[2.16] Absolute determination of σ_{tot} by A_{ss} and A_{LS} measurements.

[2.17,18,21,22] σ_{tot} absolutely determined using the lasing threshold relation; ΔN_{th} estimated from measurements of the oscillator energy or delay of the laser emission with respect to the start of the pump light.

[2.19] σ_{tot} absolutely determined using the lasing threshold relation; ΔN_{th} estimated by assuming $\Delta N_{th} = 2\,[I_2^\infty]$. The I_2^∞ concentration is measured by the iodometry method.

[2.20] $\Delta\nu$ determined over its dependence on the duration of a mode-locked oscillator pulse; data are normalized to $\alpha(n\text{-}C_3F_7I) = 14$ GHz/bar

Definition of terms: A_{ss} small signal amplification, A_{LS} large signal amplification, $R_1R_2T^2 = \exp(\sigma_{tot}\Delta N_{th}\ell)$ inversion threshold relation, R_1R_2 mirror reflectivities, T one way resonator transmission, ℓ active length.

niques are also given. In view of the accuracy of the measurements of about ± 10% the agreement is generally quite acceptable for CF_3I and the buffer gases.

Noteworthy is the discrepancy occurring for i-and n-C_3F_7I. Since the value of 14 GHz/bar for n-C_3F_7I was directly determined from a luminescence measurement [2.4], the larger values (15 GHz/bar for i-C_3F_7I and 14 GHz/bar for n-C_3F_7I) seem to be preferable.

2.1.5 Influence of Magnetic Fields

Magnetic fields can have a strong influence on the operation of an iodine laser. The following effects were observed: magnetic-field-controlled gain switch [2.23-24], magnetic field strength dependent preference of individual hyperfine components [2.25-26], polarization of the laser emission

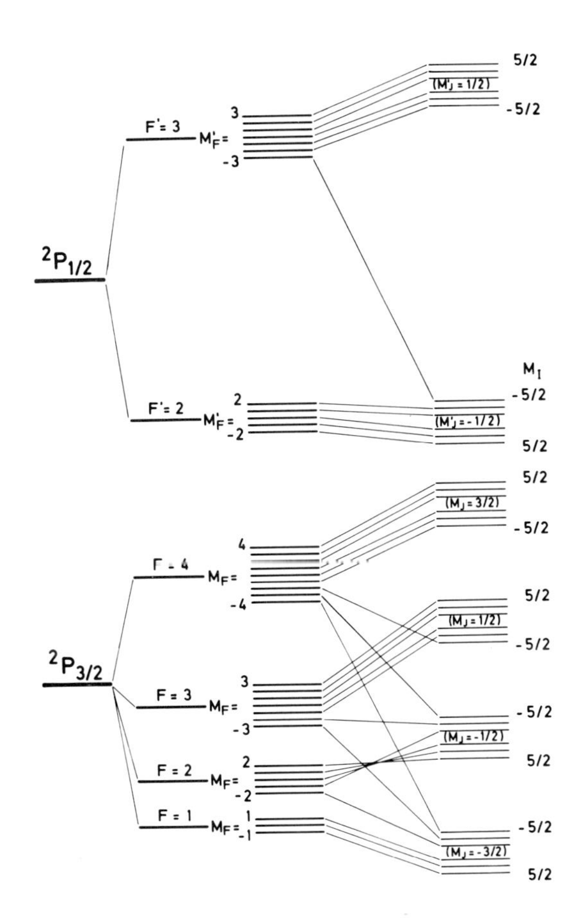

Fig. 2.4. Assignment of levels for the $^2P_{1/2}$ ground state and the $^2P_{3/2}$ first excited state of a free iodine atom ^{127}I undergoing hyperfine interaction (left), weak magnetic field interaction (centre) and strong magnetic field interaction (right)

by transverse magnetic fields, Faraday effect due to longitudinal magnetic fields [2.27] and finally continuous tunability over a spectral range of several wave numbers in cm^{-1} at very high field strengths [2.28]. Some of the phenomena mentioned are given detailed treatment in Sect. 3.1.

A term scheme of the iodine atom and its basic changes due to hyperfine interaction in an external magnetic field is shown in Fig. 2.4. Given, starting from the left, are the two shell terms characterizing the laser transition, the ground state $^2P_{3/2}$ and the excited state $^2P_{1/2}$. Proceeding to the right, we then have the familiar hyperfine splitting as a result of the interaction of the shell with the nuclear spin I = 5/2 of the only stable isotope ^{127}I. In the magnetic field the six hyperfine levels split into 36 levels altogether in keeping with their (2F+1)-fold degeneracy. On transition from the Zeeman effect (weak magnetic field) to the Back-Goudsmit effect (strong magnetic field) the number of levels does not change, but in the ground state $^2P_{3/2}$ there are several level crossings. Level crossing and changes of the good quantum numbers alter the spectrum in the magnetic field very drastically. While the unperturbed hyperfine spectrum is characterized by six separate transitions, the number of allowed transitions in the case of Zeeman effect increases to 74 lines which usually cannot be resolved owing to Doppler and pressure broadening (Sect.2.1.3).

In accordance with the two selection rules both for the total angular momentum quantum number $\Delta F = 0, \pm 1$ and the magnetic number $\Delta M_F = 0, \pm 1$, we should get 92 spectral lines by combination, but a glance at Table 2.2 of the Landé factors shows that several differently labelled transitions

Table 2.2. Landé factors of an iodine atom ^{127}I

Level	$^2P_{1/2}$	$^2P_{3/2}$
g_J	2/3	4/3
F',F	$g_{F'}$	g_F
1		-1
2	-1/9	1/9
3	1/9	7/18
4		1/2

in the magnetic field coincide energetically. This is because the variation of the transition energy in the Zeeman effect,

$$\Delta E = \mu_B(g_F M_F - g_{F'} M_{F'})H, \tag{2.11}$$

where μ_B is the Bohr magneton, g_F and $g_{F'}$ are the Landé factors in the ground and excited states, and H is the magnetic field strength, causes numerous components in the case of the 2-2 and particularly the 3-2 transition to coincide even in the presence of a magnetic field.

Table 2.3. Influence of magnetic field on $^2P_{1/2}$ - $^2P_{3/2}$ transition

Magnetic splitting range of field strengths [A/cm]	Eigenfunctions ground state	first excited state	Selection rules	Number of separated lines
Zeeman 0-400	$\langle IJFM_F\vert$	$\vert IJ'F'M_F'\rangle$	$\Delta F=0,\pm 1$ $\Delta M_F=0,\pm 1$	74
1st transition region 400-3000	$\langle IJFM_F\vert$ $\langle IJM_IM_J\vert$	$\vert IJ'F'M_F'\rangle$		
intermediate region 3000-10000	$\langle IJM_IM_J\vert$	$\vert IJ'F'M_F'\rangle$	$\Delta M=0,\pm 1$ $M=M_J+M_I$	60
2nd transition region 10000-30000	$\langle IJM_IM_J\vert$	$\vert IJ'F'M_F'\rangle$ $\vert IJ'M_I'M_J'\rangle$		
Back-Goudsmit 30000 - ∞	$\langle IJM_IM_J\vert$	$\vert IJ'M_I'M_F'\rangle$	$\Delta M_J=0,\pm 1$ $\Delta M_I=0$	36

With increasing magnetic field strength this description becomes more complex because the spectroscopic constant of the hyperfine splitting (see Sect. 2.1.1) for the ground state is rather small and, moreover, an order of magnitude smaller than that of the excited state. First of all this means that the pure Zeeman effect ($H<A_{3/2}/\mu_B \cong 600$ A/cm) only occurs up to field strengths of just a few 100 A/cm. In the excited state the hyperfine interaction does not compete with the action of an external magnetic field until field strengths $A_{1/2}/\mu_B \cong 5$ kA/cm are reached so that a pure Back-Goudsmit effect is definitely present above 30 kA/cm. Below this field strength range the system of good quantum numbers changes several times and with it the selection rules for allowed transitions. As shown in Table 2.3, a distinction can be made between three regions in which the states can be characterized by good quantum numbers and two intermediate regions characterized by strong state mixing. Each range are assigned the wave functions characterized by good quantum numbers, an estimate of the number of energetically separated transitions and the appropriate selection rules.

In the transition regions there is a pronounced increase in the number of lines because electric quadrupole transitions also exhibit high transition probabilities owing to the strong state mixing. After reasonable

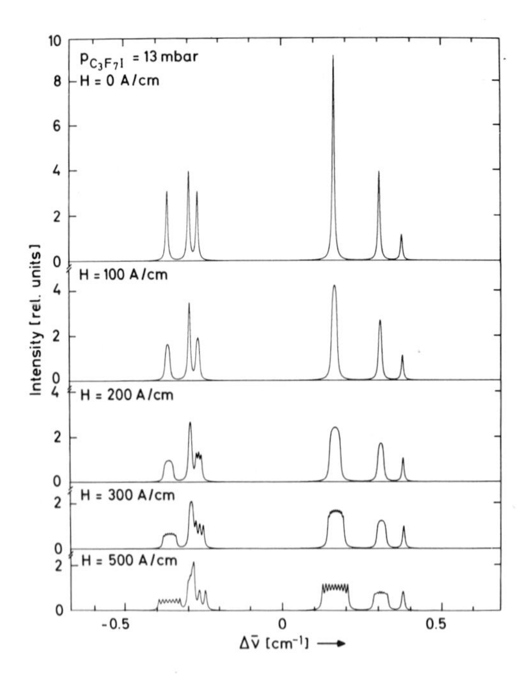

Fig. 2.5. Hyperfine spectra of an iodine atom ^{127}I in a laser medium of 13 mbar C_3F_7I subjected to different longitudinal magnetic field strengths

simplifications had been made, this behaviour was numerically simulated up to 6 kA/cm [2.29].

In spectra obtained under laser conditions many of the lines cannot be resolved because the Doppler and pressure broadening are greater than the line interval. The complicated spectra occurring in iodine lasers as a result of magnetic fields are shown in Fig. 2.5. Here a ^{127}I spectrum without field is compared with spectra having field strengths of up to 500 A/cm. It is found that at field strengths occurring in certain flash-lamp geometries the maximum of the 3-4 line may be below that of the 2-3/2-2 lines. The figure shows the influence of the magnetic field at low pressure in the active medium. With increasing gas pressure its effect is overshadowed by pressure broadening.

2.1.6 Sublevel Relaxation

Under saturation conditions the relaxation between hyperfine sublevels of a given laser level becomes an important mechanism. As will be shown in the section on pulse propagation, the relaxation time determines the energy extraction efficiency for different pulse lengths.

Hyperfine relaxation occurs almost entirely through collisions with atoms or molecules in the gas. The dominant mixing processes are, however, different for the sublevels of the ground and the excited state of the iodine atom. Whereas very efficient mixing of the ground-state sublevels results from the Van der Waals interaction in collisions with *any* particle, this is not true for the excited-state sublevels. Here the cross-sections which are involved are smaller by four to five orders of magnitude, due to the specific fine splitting ($J = 1/2$) of the $^2P_{1/2}$ state [2.30].

The various processes which can mix the excited-state sublevels faster than the Van der Waals mechanism were investigated by YUKOV [2.13]. It turned out that the most effective process is resonant energy transfer between two iodine atoms, one of them being in the ground state, the other being in the excited state. For this interaction YUKOV found a cross-section of 5.0×10^{-14} cm^2. Such a value leads to a hyperfine relaxation time of the order of several tens of ns under typical laser conditions.

As already stated, hyperfine relaxation within the lower laser level is effected with any particles in the gas. For example, the cross-section for Ar was estimated by YUKOV to be 7.0×10^{-14} cm^2 [2.13]. This cross-

-section is of the order of the cross-section for pressure broadening, and therefore the hyperfine relaxation times are of the order of the inverse linewidth.

Experimental data for the hyperfine relaxation time are only available for the upper laser level. KATULIN et al. [2.31] measured a relaxation time of 19 ns in their laser, leading to a reaction constant $k = 0.96 \pm 0.4 \times 10^{-9}\ cm^3/s$ atom for resonant energy transfer. (From YUKOV's cross-section a reaction constant of $1.5 \times 10^{-9}\ cm^3/s$ atom can be deduced).

THIEME and FILL [2.32,33] investigated the hyperfine relaxation in the upper laser level for various conditions of saturation and for various buffer gas pressures. They found that iodine in the ground state is in fact the relevant collision partner, and that the argon buffer gas pressure plays no role. For the resonant exchange transfer reaction they found a constant $k = 1.3 \pm 0.3 \times 10^{-9}\ cm^3/s$ atom, in good agreement with the theoretical value.

It follows from these results that at moderate medium linewidths $\Delta\nu \leqq 5$ GHz a laser pulse with a duration of the order of a ns extracts only the inversion energy stored in the $F = 3$ upper level when its carrier frequency is at or close to the centre frequency of the 3-4 transition.

2.2 Methods of Excitation

In this section the various methods are discussed which have been used to generate a population inversion in atomic iodine. Three different types have been distinguished: a) optical pumping, b) electron impact pumping in a discharge, and c) chemical transfer pumping.

a) The pumping scheme mostly used for pulsed operation is optical pumping by photodissociation of an iodine-atom-bearing compound,

$$RI + h\nu \xrightarrow{270\ nm} R + I(^2P_{1/2}) \ . \tag{2.12}$$

Henceforth $I(^2P_{1/2})$ will be abbreviated to I*.

b) In principle the role of the photon can also be assumed by an electron,

$$RI + e^- \quad \rightarrow \quad R + I \ \ + e^- \quad . \tag{2.13}$$

Up to now this pumping mechanism has not proved to be very efficient.

One of the main reasons is that it is hard to get a uniform stable discharge in the presence of RI molecules.

c) Chemical transfer pumping had been under discussion for several years before BENARD et al. [2.34] realized a 100-W transverse-flow oxygen-iodine chemical laser. It is based on the transfer of excitation energy,

$$O_2(^1\Delta) + I \rightleftarrows O_2(^3\Sigma) + I^* . \qquad (2.14)$$

Although only operated hitherto in the CW mode, such a laser has also some potential in pulsed operation (see Sect. 7.3). In the following discussion these three pumping methods will be dealt with in detail with special emphasis on the optical pumping process with different light sources.

2.2.1 Photodissociation of Alkyl Iodides

As early as 1938 PORRETT and GOODEVE [2.35] found during the study of the absorbed spectra of alkyl iodides that electronically excited iodine atoms are very likely produced during photolysis of CH_3I. This assumption was confirmed in 1964 by KASPAR and PIMENTEL [2.36] and in 1965 by ANDREEVA et al. [2.37] who succeeded in getting laser action by photolysis of CH_3I and CF_3I.

The absorption spectra of the various alkyl iodides are very similar. As an example Fig. 2.6 shows the absorption spectrum of CF_3I in the wavelength

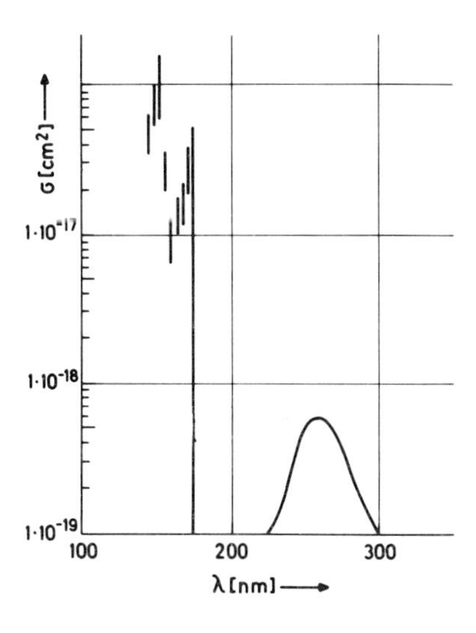

Fig. 2.6. Absorption cross-section of CF_3I between 150 and 300 nm (structure of the VUV absorption band unresolved)

region between 150 and 300 nm [2.38]. The absorption starts on the long--wavelength side with a smooth absorption band which peaks around 270 nm. The half-width (FWHM) is 37 nm. The absorption drops to practically zero at 220 nm before increasing sharply for wavelengths shorter than 180 nm. In contrast to the smooth absorption at 270 nm, the spectrum in this wavelength region is heavily structured.

The absorption at 270 nm (corresponding to a photon energy of 4.7 eV) leads to the production of I* and the radical CF_3, while the absorption below 180 nm leads to a variety of fragments, F, IF, CF [2.39]. In this context it is illustrative to note the bond strengths of the different chemical bonds in these molecules: the bond strength of the C-I binding is 2.3 eV compared with 4.5 eV for the C-C bond and 6 eV for the C-F bond. Photolysis in the region below 220 nm ≅ 5.6 eV should be avoided for laser excitation because photolysis products will cause unwanted reactions.

Successful laser experiments prompted the search for further iodine--bearing compounds which are more suitable for laser action when irradiated with light. The following alkyl iodides have been investigated in some detail:

CH_3I, CD_3I, $\underline{CF_3I}$,

CF_3CH_2I, $\underline{C_2F_5I}$, C_2H_5I,

$n\text{-}C_3H_7I$, $\underline{n\text{-}C_3F_7I}$, $\underline{i\text{-}C_3F_7I}$,

$n\text{-}C_4H_9I$, $i\text{-}C_4H_9I$, $t\text{-}C_4F_9I$.

Of these molecules only the underlined compounds have achieved practical importance. For more information see Sect. 2.3.1.

BIRICH et al. [2.40] have investigated a series of molecules containing group V elements:

$(CF_3)_2\,AsI$, $CF_3(C_2F_5)\,AsI$, $CF_3(C_3F_7)\,AsI$, $(C_2F_5)_2\,AsI$,
$(C_3F_7)_2\,AsI$,
$(CF_3)_2\,PI$, $CF_3(C_2F_5)\,PI$, $CF_3(C_3F_7)\,PI$, $(C_2F_5)_2\,PI$,
$(C_3F_7)_2\,PI$,
$CF_3\,CH_3\,PI$, $CF_3\,PI(CN)$, $CF_3(CF_2Cl)(CFH)\,PI$, F_3PI, OPF_2I,
and $(CF_3)_2\,Sb\,I$.

The absorption bands of these molecules are very similar to those of alkyl iodides. The maximum of the I* producing band is at around 280 nm for nearly all these compounds ($\pm$ 5 nm). In addition, they all have a much larger absorption cross-section, 3×10^{-18} cm^2 versus about 6×10^{-19} cm^2 for alkyl iodides (see Table 2.4). However, there is no serious competitor to the alkyl iodides among the substances containing a group V element. Besides being more difficult to synthesize, they show strong thermal decomposition when irradiated with high light intensities.

HOFFMANN and LEONE [2.41] have investigated HgI_2 as a source of I*. HgI_2 produces I* when irradiated with light at a wavelength of around 270 nm. The maximum absorption cross-section is 1.5×10^{-17} cm^2. This system affords a very exciting advantage: it is totally reversible, which means that $I(^2P_{3/2})$ will react back to HgI_2 with the HgI radical. The high deactivation rate of I* by the parent molecule HgI_2 ($k = 4.5 \times 10^{-10}$ cm^3/s molecule) limits the pumping time. Ordinary flashlamps can probably not be used, but laser excitation seems entirely feasible. For instance, pumping with a KrF excimer laser affords the possibility of constructing an iodine oscillator with a high repetition rate.

Another candidate for a reversible iodine laser was investigated by DAVIS [2.42]. I_2 molecules were dissociated with a dye laser at a wavelength of around 497 nm yielding I and I*. Because of the degeneracy of the upper and lower laser levels (Sect. 2.1.1) population inversion was obtained. Although the efficiency of this laser was very low - 10^{-5} relative to the dye laser energy - it is an interesting type of sealed-off iodine laser with high repetition rate.

With the exception of I_2 and HgI_2, which are of no practical importance for high-power iodine lasers, there are no detailed spectroscopic data available on potential curves of the parent molecules. As already mentioned, the only substances of practical importance are the alkyl iodides: $n\text{-}C_3F_7I$, $i\text{-}C_3F_7I$, C_2F_5I and CF_3I. Their quantum yield for I* production has been measured by several authors (see Table 2.4). The quantum yield for all compounds is close to unity. All others substances have lower yields and less favourable kinetic properties. This explains why only the afore--mentioned fluorinated compounds are used in practice.

The location and width of the absorption band of the iodides plays a role in determining the efficiency of the laser. Before the possibilities of generating light in the spectral range concerned with here are discussed, a method which allows the absorption band to be increased and shifted should be mentioned. PUMMER et al. [2.43] have irradiated the alkyl iodide CF_3I with CO_2 laser radiation, thus populating the ν_1 vibrational mode of the molecule. Vibrational excitation can alter the absorption spectrum by the following three effects: a) molecular symmetry changes, which can cause vibronically allowed transitions; b) the Franck-Condon factors change, thus allowing transitions to different portions of the excited-state surface (broadening of the band); c) a red shift which is directly related to the energy of the vibrationally excited state. First experiments did in fact reveal that vibrationally excited CF_3I showed absorption at longer wavelengths than the unexcited species. A continuation of these experiments by PADRICK [2.44] confirmed the results in [2.43]. Increases of the FWHM of the absorption spectrum of up to a factor of 2.2 were observed. However, it was also found that the broadening is accompanied by an appreciable amount of decomposition of CF_3I leading to the formation of ground-state iodine atoms. Thus, the inversion is greatly reduced. If the decomposition problem could somehow be avoided, this technique would be an attractive way to improve the efficiency of the iodine laser.

2.2.2 Flashlamp Technology

The discussion of the various iodides has shown that the most suitable iodides are CF_3I, C_2F_5I and C_3F_7I. They have an absorption band near 280 nm which is 35 to 45 nm broad (FWHM) (Table 2.4). The maximum absorption cross-section is roughly 6×10^{-19} cm^2. The quantum yield for producing I^* is nearly unity throughout the whole absorption band. For efficient pumping of the iodine laser the light source has to have a high efficiency in this spectral region. For comparison, a black-body radiator of 10 000 K has its maximum brightness at 290 nm. Compared with neodymium or ruby laser pump bands, the light source has to be much "hotter". Another difficulty in building a suitable light source for the iodine laser is that the light flash has to be very short in time. This is due to the fact that the flash causes a shock wave in the laser medium, originating from the laser tube wall. This shock wave normally travels slightly faster than the speed of sound and seriously disturbs the optical quality of the gas behind the shock front. Good laser beam quality can only be achieved with unperturbed gas. This shock wave problem, which will be discussed in more detail in Chap. 4, limits the time duration of the flash to ≤ 20 μs, depending on the size of the laser tube.

Several methods have been used to realize an efficient light source for the iodine laser:

a) flashlamps,
b) open high-current discharges,
c) surface sparks,
d) multiple-arc sources,
e) laser-produced plasmas in the laser gas, and
f) excimer light sources.

a) The light sources most commonly used are flashlamps. The technology of flashlamps has been well established for several years because they are the main pumping light sources for ruby, Nd glass and dye lasers. The special requirements for pumping a high-power iodine laser (short wavelength, short pulse length, high power density) made it necessary to develop a special type of flashlamp. The lamps available for pumping other lasers are not directly suitable for the iodine laser. Extensive studies of flashlamp parameters have only been conducted for long pulse lengths (≧ 200 μs) in support of the big Nd glass laser programs, especially at Lawrence Livermore Laboratory [2.45,46]. Unfortunalty the relations found between the various lamp parameters for these long-time lamps cannot be directly applied to the short-pulse lamps. No computer simulations are thus available for the current, impedance and output radiation of short-pulse flashlamps in given spectral bands. Attention is therefore confined here to some experimental results on lamps developed at MPQ Garching [2.47].

The main questions concerning flashlamps are:

1) efficiency of the lamp in the spectral range of interest, and
2) the lifetime of the lamps under high loading conditions.

The flashlamps mostly used in the Garching iodine laser systems, have an active length of up to 100 cm. The envelope of these lamps is a quartz tube with an inner diameter of up to 2.5 cm. It turned out that of the rare gases xenon shows the best efficiency. In contrast to lamps for other laser systems, the pressure of the xenon gas has to be rather low (about 40 mbar) to achieve best results, for pumping time durations ≦ 20 μs. Above a power load of 1 MW/cm^3 (within the 20-μs duration) the efficiency is only a weak function of the input energy. The absolute value of the lamp efficiency (defined as the energy emitted by the lamp suitable for pumping per energy stored in the capacitors) is hard to determine because several effects influence the measurements. If the number of iodine molecules formed from photolytically generated iodine atoms is compared with the lamp energy, not only the detailed kinetic processes but also the influence of the reflectors have to be taken into account. A fair measure seems to be the following procedure: if the oscillator efficiencies η (oscillator output energy per stored electric energy) of the various devices are compared, the maximum attainable efficiency will set a lower limit to the lamp efficiency. The oscillator efficiency measured with these lamps was between 1.1% and 1.4% [2.48,49] for a flashlamp-pumped iodine laser. In [2.48] the flashlamps were located outside the laser tube whereas in [2.49] the flashlamp was embedded in the laser medium. In both cases the alkyl iodide pressure was so high that the laser medium was optically thick with respect to the pumping radiation. Under these conditions η can be represented by $\eta = \eta_\ell \cdot \eta_q \cdot \eta_{tr} \cdot \eta_c$ where η_ℓ denotes the lamp efficiency, $\eta_q = (h\nu_{laser}/h\nu_{pump}) = 0.21$ the quantum efficiency, η_{tr} the electrical losses in the discharge circuit and η_c the reflector losses. Assuming $\eta_{tr} = 0.85$ for both configurations and $\eta_c = 0.75$ for [2.48] and $\eta_c = 1$ for [2.49], a lamp efficiency η_ℓ of about 8% is obtained in both cases. This means that 8% of the energy stored in the capacitor banks is transformed into light suitable for the iodine laser.

If the xenon plasma radiated like a black body with a temperature of nearly 10 000 K, about 10% of the radiation would go into the spectral band of interest. This means that these flashlamps already operate near the maximum efficiency, taking into account thermodynamic equilibrium of the xenon plasma. Further major improvements in the lamp efficiency can therefore only be obtained with line source radiators. Normally, the spectra of xenon flashlamps are composed of a continuum and a line spectrum. There is some discussion whether the efficiency can be improved by doping the gas with substances which radiate especially in the wavelength regime of interest. The only successful experiments were published by GUSINOV [2.50]. He reported that adding some powdered zinc (0.15 grams to a 70-cm^3 lamp filled with 27 mbar xenon) increases the efficiency by a factor of two to three. Unfortunately, after several shots considerable degeneration takes place, probably owing to "clean-up" of the zinc. This "clean-up" problem was solved by PALMER [2.51] for the case of Te-doped flashlamps. The results of this work suggest that while metal additives do enhance the near-UV-output radiation, the degree of enhancement is such that they do not warrant further investigation at this time with regard to application of pumping an iodine laser.

Experiments have shown that the lifetime of a flashlamp is strongly related to its explosion energy because according to a widely accepted law the number of shots n is an exponential function of the ratio of the explosion energy E_{exp} of a lamp to its input energy E according to $n = (E_{exp}/E)^m$ where m is about 7. If this ratio is unity, the shot number is just one shot, while at a ratio of 5 the shot number is $\sim 10^5$ shots. In a test series NAKAMURA [2.47] found that for the Garching lamp the explosion limit can be estimated by the following formula:

$$E_{exp} = k\ell d(T_p)^{1/2}[J], \tag{2.15}$$

where k is a numerical factor, ℓ the length and d the inner diameter of the lamp, both in cm, and T_p is the discharge time in seconds. The type of lamp with a fast UV-radiation output ($t_{rise} = 4$ µs) is operated at small xenon pressures, typically around 40 mbar. In this case the pressure dependance of E_{exp} is weak and thus omitted in (2.15). The numerical value of k for 2-mm wall thickness is 1.8×10^4, and for 3 mm it is 2.6×10^4. A 3-mm tube with a diameter of 1.8 cm and a length of 90 cm thus has an explosion limit of 19 kJ. A lifetime of several thousand shots is therefore expected for an energy load of 5 kJ within 20 µs.

In conclusion, it can be stated that flashlamp technology has developed to such a state that lamps are available which provide the UV-light required for excitation of the iodine laser with an efficiency of at least 7% at power loads of 1 MW/cm^3. The pulse length is up to 20 µs at a lifetime of several thousand shots.

b) At the Lebedev Institute another light source for pumping the iodine laser was developed: open high-current discharges [2.52,53]. These are known to be high-power light sources, particularly in the UV spectral range. The brightness temperature can reach 40 000 to 50 000 K for a sufficiently high current [2.54]. Normally, the electric explosion of a thin metallic wire spanning a distance of 1.5 m in the laser gas itself is used to initiate a long cylindrical discharge. The development of the discharge occurs in two steps: firstly, the wire sublimates under the influence of the initial current and forms a high-density gas column; secondly, this gas expands and the main discharge takes place if the voltage is high enough. During the discharge a shock wave is formed which runs into the ambient gas. The main advantage of this light source is the high pump power which can be achieved. At the Lebedev Institute energies in excess of 200 kJ have been discharged in one device within 60 μs. The reported laser efficiency is 0.6%, comparing the laser energy and the energy stored in the capacitors. The laser construction is simple because it consists only of a metal tube with a metal wire spanning the axis. Besides these technical advantages, open high-current discharges entail some severe problems. The laser gas itself is used up very quickly because the molecules are destroyed either by thermal effects or by electron impact in the discharge region. In the shock front the density of the laser gas can reach high values, thus causing high inversion densities, which can in turn give raise to parasitic oscillations. The strong magnetic fields originating from the high current density considerably alter the stimulated emission cross-section. The circuit inductance cannot be made as small as in the case of flashlamps so that the UV-pulse rise time will generally be $\geqq$ 20 μs. The repetition rate is limited by the replacement time for the exploding wire. In the system now used, the laser chamber normally has to be opened to replace the wire, thus limiting the repetition rate to a few shots per day. In principle, however, automatic replacement systems are possible. To sum up, open discharges offer a very powerful and inexpensive UV-light source. These advantages are balanced by the limited efficiency, the strong shock waves, the high inductance and the low repetition rate.

c) BEVERLY et al. [2.55] have made an extensive study on another type of open discharge: surface-spark discharges. In their experiment a discharge was formed between two electrodes mounted on a surface. The basic idea is that the surface material will partly evaporate under the influence of the discharge plasma. The evaporated material will then radiate in highly broadened lines, leading to high efficiencies. BEVERLY et al. used a variety of substances for the substrate (BN, Al_2O_3, ZrO_2, ZnO, $BaTiO_3$, ZnO x Al_2O_3 and Cr_2O_3 x Al_2O_3) at different channel energy depositions (10 to 100 J/cm). The efficiency depends on the ambient gas pressure. The best results were obtained with Cr_2O_3 x Al_2O_3 immersed in Ar gas at several bar. The maximum reported efficiency was 9.4% $\pm$ 1.1% into the 250- to 290-nm pump band of the iodine laser. These measurements were not performed in real laser devices but with calibrated films. The advantages and disadvantages of these light sources can be judged to be very similar to the exploding wire devices with the exception that higher repetition rates are possible with spark gaps.

d) Multiple-arc sources were already used in 1969 by GENSEL et al. [2.56] to pump an iodine laser. A spectroscopic study of these light sources was performed by BEVERLY et al. [2.57] by putting a series of 34 coaxial-geometry spark plugs into the laser gas, which was mainly composed of He or Ar and SF_6 together with a few per cent of i-C_3F_7I. Their best results yielded an estimated efficiency of 3% to 4% for the radiation into the interesting pump band. These results are estimated from film exposures and are not obtained in laser devices.

e) SILFVAST et al. [2.58] have investigated CO_2-laser-produced plasma as light source. They focused a CO_2 laser beam of 2.75 J in front of an aluminium reflector to produce a bright xenon plasma. By comparing the laser energy they found that the laser-produced plasma has a light output at least three times that of an ordinary xenon flashlamp powered with the same energy density. Using a CO_2 laser with an efficiency of 30% would thus yield an overall efficiency comparable to that of flashlamps. But these light sources would offer higher repetition rates and higher pump rates together with shorter pumping times which would be interesting in, for instance, decoupling amplifiers in a laser chain. Unfortunately, no other groups have taken up this very interesting concept.

f) Recent experiments have shown that rare-gas halogen excimers and diatomic halogen molecules are efficient, relatively narrow-band radiators in the spectral region between 190 and 350 nm. The most attractive systems are KrF, XeBr and XeCl, which emit in the absorption band of the alkyl iodides [2.59]. The radiation of these excimers can either be used as a fluorescence source or as a laser. Fluorescence pumping was realized at Lawrence Livermore Laboratory [2.60,61] where gain at 1.3 μm was demonstrated in C_3F_7I dissociated by fluorescence light from XeBr. Pumping by means of laser light was investigated by FILL et al. [2.62]. An iodine oscillator filled with C_3F_7I was successfully operated. Either a KrF or a XeCl laser was used as a pump source. In this paper it was also shown that at least up to pumping levels of 50 MW/cm^2 no thermal decomposition or multiphoton dissociation of the C_3F_7I molecule occurs at pressures up to 400 mbar.

From a practical point of view pumping of an iodine amplifier by excimer laser radiation is to be preferred over pumping by excimer fluorescence. An efficient coupling of the pump light to the alkyl iodide together with the requirement of a spatially homogeneous inversion profile is difficult to realize in the case of fluorescence since the light is emitted into a solid angle of 4 π and, moreover, excimer devices are rather voluminous.

When operated in the form of an electric discharge an excimer laser can deliver an output pulse of up to a few joules of energy and some 10-ns duration at a repetition rate of up to 1 kHz. This makes it an attractive pump source for the preamplifiers in an amplifier chain since a short UV laser pulse can help to increase the threshold for the occurrence of parasitic oscillations resulting from amplifier coupling. Another interesting application of these excimer lasers is to use them as a pump source for iodine oscillators delivering temporally smooth pulses of a few ns duration at a high repetition rate [2.62].

For output energies in the kJ range, electron-beam-pumped systems have to be used. Their efficiency is expected to be quite high, of the order of 10% or even somewhat more (flashlamps ~ 7%). The repetition rate will be about 1/60 Hz and thus comparable to that of flashlamps. Since, however, such systems will not be available in the near future and are rather complex, they represent an inferior alternative to flashlamps as a pump source for large iodine amplifiers.

To summarize light pump technology, it can be stated that with respect to efficiency, scalability and repetition rate flashlamps currently are the most suitable light sources for an iodine laser system. Only for small amplifiers and high-repetition-rate lasers with small energies, such as oscillators for large laser systems, are some of the other pumping schemes described above interesting alternatives, especially the excimer lasers driven by an electric discharge.

2.2.3 Excitation in a Direct Discharge

As already pointed out, pumping of the iodine laser can be accomplished not only with photons but also with electrons. In 1974 ZALESSKII and IVANOV [2.63,64] proposed the possibility of excited iodine atom production by electron impact in a glow discharge. In 1975 PLEASANCE and WEAVER observed for the first time iodine laser emission in a transverse discharge [2.65]. They used a CO_2 laser discharge device preionized with UV light which was emitted by sparks behind one of the electrodes. The discharge volume was 2 x 2 x 50 cm^3 and the applied voltage was varied between 10 and 35 kV. The gas was composed of 93 mbar N_2 and of up to 1.3 mbar CF_3I. The driving capacitor had a capacity of 20 nF. Above 1.3 mbar CF_3I, the discharge tended to be unstable during a discharge time of approximately

150 ns. The unstable character was believed due to the electron affinity of CF_3I. Although the measured laser energy was rather small (0.3 mJ), these experiments demonstrated that the electron impact dissociation of alkyl iodide molecules leads to the formation of excited iodine atoms. PLEASANCE and WEAVER observed a delayed laser emission, which they attributed to removal of ground-state iodine atoms by chemical kinetics. These ground--state iodine atoms react faster than the excited iodine atoms thus leading to inversion. A more detailed understanding of the processes in a discharge was gained by the investigations of WONG and BEVERLY [2.66,67]. In a similar device they used a mixture of $i\text{-}C_3F_7I$ and He at a total pressure of 93 mbar (maximum alkyl iodide gas pressure 1.3 mbar) and obtained a laser energy of about 0.5 mJ. No delay of the emission was observed in these experiments. The authors developed a theoretical model from which they concluded that the fraction of excited iodine atoms $I^*/(I^*+I)$ amounts to about 0.5. This means that equal portions of excited- and ground-state iodine atoms are formed by the electron impact process. It is then evident that this excitation process is basically very inefficient and has to rely on "good" kinetics of the gas mixture. Nevertheless, this pumping scheme may be attractive but further experiments need to be performed to judge its limitations properly.

2.2.4 Chemical Excitation

While the photolytic and electron impact pumping of the iodine laser are based on the dissociation of alkyl iodide molecules, chemical excitation starts from a completely different scheme. Here excited iodine atoms I^* are generated as a result of a collisional energy transfer from an excited oxygen molecule $O_2(^1\Delta)$ to an iodine atom I in the ground state according to

$$O_2(^1\Delta) + I \rightleftarrows O_2(^3\Sigma) + I^* \quad . \tag{2.16}$$

The corresponding energy levels are shown in Fig. 2.7. Since the interaction (2.16) is fast both in the forward and backward directions (k_{eq} = 8×10^{-11} cm^3/s molecule), it reaches equilibrium even in the presence of other fast reactions. The equilibrium constant k_{eq} defined by

$$k_{eq} = \frac{[O_2(^3\Sigma)][I^*]}{[O_2(^1\Delta)][I]} \tag{2.17}$$

- square brackets indicate concentrations - has a value of 2.9 at room temperature. Thus, an iodine inversion $[I^*] - 1/2\ [I] > 0$ exists whenever $[O_2(^1\Delta)]\ /\ [O_2(^3\Sigma)] > 0.17$. Because of the low value of k_{eq}, most of the energy of the chemical system is carried by $O_2(^1\Delta)$. Efficient energy extraction therefore requires a multiple energy transfer from $O_2(^1\Delta)$ molecules to iodine atoms.

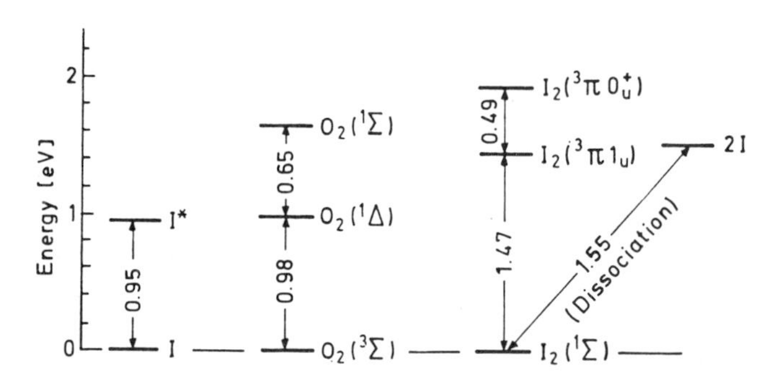

Fig. 2.7. Relevant energy states of I, O_2 and I_2 in the chemical pumping scheme

The practical application of this I* producing reaction requires an efficient chemical $O_2(^1\Delta)$ generator and the dissociation of molecular iodine to 2 I by $O_2(^1\Delta)$ molecules. McDERMOTT et al. [2.68] finally succeeded in 1977 at the Air Force Weapons Laboratory (Kirtland, NM, USA) in getting an iodine laser to operate (CW) on the basis of this transfer scheme. While this first chemically excited iodine laser had only a few mW output power, the same group scaled up their experiments and obtained several 100 W some months later [2.34]; another group achieved 10 W [2.69].

The most important component in these devices is the $O_2(^1\Delta)$ generator. A Cl_2 stream is bubbled through a basic solution of H_2O_2 and NaOH. $O_2(^1\Delta)$ is evolved into the gas phase by the overall reaction

$$Cl_2 + H_2O_2 + 2NaOH \rightarrow O_2(^1\Delta) + 2H_2O + 2NaCl\ . \tag{2.18}$$

In the experiments reported in [2.34,68,69] about 40% of the oxygen molecules formed are in the $O_2(^1\Delta)$ state; in a more recent investigation [2.70], approximately 100% were achieved. The generator effluent passes through a liquid-nitrogen-cooled trap to remove H_2O and excess Cl_2. Just in front of the laser cavity the $O_2(^1\Delta)$ gas is mixed with an I_2/Ar gas stream. Excited iodine atoms are formed in the reaction zone and transported to the resonator, the axis of which is perpendicular to the flow direction. In [2.68] the active laser tube diameter was 15 cm; the laser emitted more than 100 W over periods of up to 3 min.

Until recently the dissociation of I_2 in the chemically pumped iodine laser was believed to occur in a two step process according to

$$O_2(^1\Delta) + O_2(^1\Delta) \rightarrow O_2(^1\Sigma) + O_2(^3\Sigma) \tag{2.19}$$

and

$$O_2(^1\Sigma) + I_2 \rightarrow 2\,I + O_2(^3\Sigma) \quad . \tag{2.20}$$

This sequence was suggested by DERWENT and THRUSH [2.71] in 1972. Although this collisional dissociation of I_2 has been directly observed [2.72] it is *not* the most important source of iodine atoms in the oxygen-iodine laser since the rate constant of reaction (2.20) is too low [2.72,73] to account for the efficient dissociation of I_2. Moreover, $O_2(^1\Sigma)$ is strongly quenched by H_2O [2.73,74]; experiments without any $O_2(^1\Sigma)$ due to the presence of H_2O yielded output powers similar to the case without any H_2O.

What other mechanism is then responsible for the buildup of I atoms is presently a matter of speculation. It can only be stated that the overall reaction given by

$$I_2 + nO_2(^1\Delta) \rightarrow 2I + (n-2)O_2(^1\Delta) + 2O_2(^3\Sigma) \tag{2.21}$$

is relatively fast and that the intermediate steps are as yet unknown.

The chemical pumping scheme as outlined above is well suited for CW operation. It has also some potential for energy storage application, e.g. as a pulsed device for plasma experiments. However, in this case the energy stored in the system can only be extracted via a multiple pass technique because most of the extractable energy is deposited in the $O_2(^1\Delta)$ molecules and not in the I* atoms. Theoretical investigations on the feasibility of such an iodine laser system have been reported in [2.70,75]. Between 10 and 20 passes through an amplifier have been envisaged as being necessary in order to extract a large fraction ($\geqq$ 80%) of the energy stored in the oxygen molecules and iodine atoms. High overall efficiencies are claimed, 6% with the inclusion of the regeneration of the parent molecules in [2.70] and more than 10% in [2.75] without regeneration.

2.3 Chemical Kinetics of the Photodissociation Iodine Laser

In this section all the chemical reactions occurring during and after the photolysis of alkyl iodides and influencing the laser performance will be treated. Firstly the physical properties of these molecules which are essential in this context, i.e. absorption spectrum and quantum yield $f = N_{I*}/(N_{I*}+N_I)$ (N is the number density), will be presented, followed by some considerations concerning the relative performance of the perfluoroalkyl iodides for the two kinds of laser operation - oscillator mode and amplifier mode. Next the regeneration capability of perfluoroalkyl iodides, i.e. their multiple-shot performance, is dealt with. Kinetic studies are then reviewed which present the chemical reactions considered essential and the pertinent rate constants. Finally, inversion losses due to quenching of excited iodine atoms are discussed, an important issue with regard to the length of the pump pulse.

2.3.1 Alkyl Iodides

As already outlined in Sect. 2.2, only the perfluoroalkyl iodides such as CF_3I, C_2F_5I, i-C_3F_7I and n-C_3F_7I have gained practical importance for the iodine laser. Their superiority over the hydrated alkyl iodides such as CH_3I, C_2H_5I, n-C_4H_9I is based upon a larger fractional yield f of excited iodine atoms following the broadband UV photolysis [2.76-78] and upon rate constants for collisional deactivation of excited iodine atoms being smaller by two to three orders of magnitude [2.5, 79-83]. These two facts explain why under otherwise equal conditions the perfluoroalkyl iodides yield a considerably larger laser energy output and are better suited to energy storage (amplifier mode of operation) than the non-fluorinated alkyl iodides.

With respect to the compounds containing the group V atoms [2.40], the situation is not quite clear since the available information is insufficient to make a comparative study; e.g., there are no data for the deactivation rate constants. Moreover, the question of the possible toxicity of these compounds or the products originating from their photolysis has not been dealt with. Furthermore, as already pointed out in Sect. 2.2, they seem to show appreciable thermal decomposition when irradiated with strong pump light. In view of these uncertainties, only the perfluoroalkyl iodides are dealt with in the following.

Table 2.4 summarizes some essential properties of the perfluoroalkyl iodides mostly used at present. The first three columns refer to the absorption spectrum (λ_{max} is the wavelength at the absorption peak, σ_{max} the cross-section at λ_{max}, and $\Delta\lambda_{FWHM}$ the full absorption bandwidth at half maximum) and can be used for determining the fraction of the pump light absorbed in the laser medium. Since the absorption peaks are quite close together, λ_{max} is not relevant in this context.

For broadband photolysis the pump energy e_{abs} deposited in the laser medium is usually dependent on σ_{max}. If, however, inversion profiles of equal shape are compared, only the product $\sigma_{max}N_{RI}d$ (d is the tube diameter) is significant so that e_{abs} is then only proportional to $\Delta\lambda_{FWHM}$.

For the stored energy (or inversion) the quantum yield f of the excited iodine atoms I^* is the most important quantity. As can be seen from Table 2.4 the values quoted in the literature do not vary a great deal with the exceptions of $i\text{-}C_3F_7I$ and $t\text{-}C_4F_9I$.[1]

For the assessment of the molecules listed in Table 2.4 the rate constants of three processes in which they are involved also have to be considered. These are the collisional deacitivation of I^* by the parent molecule RI itself according to $I^* + RI \rightarrow I + RI$, the recombination process $R + I \rightarrow RI$ and the dimerization process $2R \rightarrow R_2$. The pertaining rate constants k_{RI}, k_R and k_D are given in Table 2.5.

2.3.2 Medium Comparison

The data pertaining to the perfluoroalkyl iodides presented in Tables 2.4,5 are sufficient for comparing their relative performances in a photodissociation laser system. However, the oscillator and amplifier modes of operation have to be distinguished. The aim in both cases is to find the

[1] According to [2.88], f of $i\text{-}C_3F_7I$ (integrated over pump band) is much lower than f of $n\text{-}C_3F_7I$. This should result in a much poorer laser performance of $i\text{-}C_3F_7I$ compared to that of $n\text{-}C_3F_7I$, which has not been confirmed experimentally. Both compounds provide nearly equal performances [2.22, 84]. Moreover, at 266 nm the data of [2.87, 88] and [2.86] can be directly compared with respect to $n\text{-}C_3F_7I$, $f = 0.86$ versus $f = 0.98$. These arguments make the f value for $i\text{-}C_3F_7I$ given in [2.87, 88] questionable. The discrepancy regarding $t\text{-}C_4F_9I$ is presently difficult to explain due to the lack of sufficient experimental data.

Table 2.4. Absorption spectrum data and quantum yield of the perfluoroalkyl iodides CF_3I, C_2F_5I, $n\text{-}C_3F_7I$, $i\text{-}C_3F_7I$ and $t\text{-}C_4F_9I$

PER-FLUORO-ALKYL IODIDE	ABSORPTION SPECTRUM DATA				QUANTUM YIELD $f = \frac{n_I^*}{n_I^* + n_I}$		
	λ_{max} [nm]	$\Delta\lambda_{FWHM}$ [nm]	$\sigma_{max} \cdot 10^{19}$ [cm^2]	Ref.	f	Comment	Ref.
CF_3I	266	37	5.4	2.22, 2.84, 2.85	0.91 ± 0.03	averaged over absorpt. spectrum	2.76, 2.77
					0.91 ± 0.005	266 nm	2.86
					$0.98^{+0.02}_{-0.09}$	averaged over abs. spectrum	2.88
	266	35	5.6	2.38	0.75 ± 0.05	248nm	2.38
					0.83 ± 0.05	308nm	2.38
C_2F_5I	266	40	6.5	2.22, 2.84	> 0.98	averaged ov. abs. spectr.	2.76, 2.77
					$0.96^{+0.04}_{-0.09}$	averaged ov. abs. spectr.	2.87
	267	38	6.4	2.38	1.01 ± 0.05	248 nm	2.38
					1.04 ± 0.05	308 nm	2.38
$n\text{-}C_3F_7I$	270	43	7.1	2.22, 2.84	> 0.99	averaged ov. abs. spectr.	2.76, 2.77
					$0.88^{+0.02}_{-0.09}$	averaged ov. abs. spectr.	2.88, 2.87
	270	41	7.8	2.38	0.97–0.99	266 nm	2.86
					1.03 ± 0.05	248nm	2.38
					0.96 ± 0.05	308nm	2.38
$i\text{-}C_3F_7I$	273	43	6.2	2.22, 2.84, 2.85	0.90 ± 0.02	averaged ov. abs. spectr.	2.76, 2.77
					$0.52 + 0.09$	averaged ov. abs. spectr.	2.88, 2.87
	274	42	6.0	2.38	0.93 ± 0.05	248 nm	2.38
					1.01 ± 0.05	308nm	2.38
$t\text{-}C_4F_9I$	288	50	6.0	2.38	0.877 ± 0.01	266 nm	2.86
					0.40 ± 0.04	averaged over abs. spectrum	2.78

Measurement techniques employed in the quoted references:

2.76,77 Flash photolysis using a krypton lamp with a continuous spectrum
2.86 Laser photolysis at 266 nm using a frequency-quadrupled Nd laser
2.78,87,88 Photochemical method based on NOCl
2.38 Laser photolysis using an KrF-and XeCl excimer laser at 248 and 308 nm

compound yielding the maximum energy output for the same electrical energy stored in the capacitor banks at an equal homogeneity level ($\sigma_{max}N_{RI}d \sim 2$ for a flat profile) and for single-shot operation (always a fresh filling). Laser medium regeneration aspects will not be considered in this context since they might lead to different conclusions.

Oscillator Mode of Operation. This mode is characterized by the de-excitation of excited iodine atoms by induced emission. In the case of *fast* flash photolysis (pumping time less than 20 μs), the quenching of the excited iodine atoms by the parent molecule is not effective and therefore does not need to be considered. Of relevance then are only the width of the absorption band, the quantum yield f and the chemical behaviour characterized by the recombination and dimerization processes. These processes are briefly considered in the next paragraph.

The output energy E_{out} of an oscillator is given by the expression $E_{out}=f_{out}f_{Deg}(E_{st}-E_{th})$ where E_{st} is the energy stored in the excited iodine atoms and E_{th} the threshold energy; f_{out} is the coupling factor of the cavity and is unity in the case of no internal losses; f_{Deg} characterizes the fraction of $E_{st}-E_{th}$ which is convertible to laser radiation. When there is no recombination of ground-state iodine atoms with radicals to form the parent molecule, f_{Deg} is given by $(1+g_u/g_\ell)^{-1} = 2/3$ where $g_u = 12$ and $g_\ell = 24$ are the degeneracy factors of the upper and lower laser levels. If, however, the situation is such that all ground--state iodine atoms can find a radical to recombine to form RI (full recombination), f_{Deg} becomes unity corresponding formally to $g_\ell = \infty$. The actual situation lies between these two limiting cases as analyzed in [2.89]. There the following expression was derived: $f_{Deg}=(2/3)[1+(1/2)\exp(-k_D/k_R)]$, which describes the cases of no recombination, $k_D >> k_{RI}$, and full recombination, $k_D << k_{RI}$, correctly. For all the compounds listed in Table 2.4, $f_{Deg} \geqq 0.9$.

One can define a figure of merit for comparing the various perfluoroalkyl iodides with respect to a maximum value of E_{out} at an equal homogeneity level. For negligible threshold energy, this figure is shown in [2.89] to be proportional to the expression $\Delta\lambda_{FWHM}(f_{Deg}+f-1) \cong \Delta\lambda_{FWHM}f_{Deg}f$ (f_{Deg} and f are close to unity). According to Tables 2.4,5 the figure of merit has the lowest value for CF_3I (29 nm) and the largest for t-C_4F_9I (44 nm); n-C_3F_7I and i-C_3F_7I show a similar behaviour, 37 and 38 nm. This finding is experimentally confirmed [2.89] except in the case of t-C_4F_9I, for which no measurements are available.

Amplifier Mode of Operation. The main concern here is the inversion available at the release time of the pulse to be amplified. Under the constraint of an equal homogeneity level for all compounds it is simply proportional to the product $\Delta\lambda_{FWHM}f$ [2.89]. In this case the *fast* recombination process $R + I \rightarrow RI$ does not play any role. Only the deactivation capability of the laser medium caused either by the parent molecule itself, the buffer gas or impurities may become important. These quenching processes can, however, usually be neglected in the case of *fast* flash photolysis so that for the amplifier mode of operation the figure of merit is simply $\Delta\lambda_{FWHM}f$. According to Table 2.4 it has its maximum value of 44 nm for t-C_4F_9I, followed by 42 nm for n-C_3F_7I, 39 nm for i-C_3F_7I, and 34 nm for CF_3I.

In both the amplifier and oscillator modes of operation, t-C_4F_9I is thus the best-performing compound. In the amplifier mode the differences are, however, less pronounced; here, n-C_3F_7I and i-C_3F_7I are also a good choice, especially in connection with a closed loop system [2.90] for which t-C_4F_9I is not as appropriate because it does not have a liquid phase at or below room temperature. Because of this fact it is also difficult to purify.

2.3.3 Regeneration of the Laser Medium

In the preceding section the problem of medium selection was treated with the intention of achieving maximum energy output. This generally requires laser medium replacement after each shot. If this is not possible, i.e. when the same mixture is flashed several times, the regeneration capability of the laser medium becomes an important issue, especially with respect to a sealed-off operation. Until recently, this subject has found relatively little attention in the literature. There are a few experiments which will be reviewed in the following and from which some conclusions can be drawn regarding laser operation without medium exchange.

In Fig. 2.8 the multiple-shot performance of a single i-C_3F_7I filling is shown, both for the oscillator and amplifier modes of operation. A quasi-equilibrium state appears to be possible after 50 to 100 shots.

Similar results have also been obtained for the other perfluoroalkyl iodides CF_3I, C_2F_5I and n-C_3F_7I [2.22, 84]. Since they show a larger decrease of performance after multiple shots compared with i-C_3F_7I they are not considered further here.

The fraction of the initial value of the output energy which can be finally reached in the quasi-equilibrium state depends on a variety of

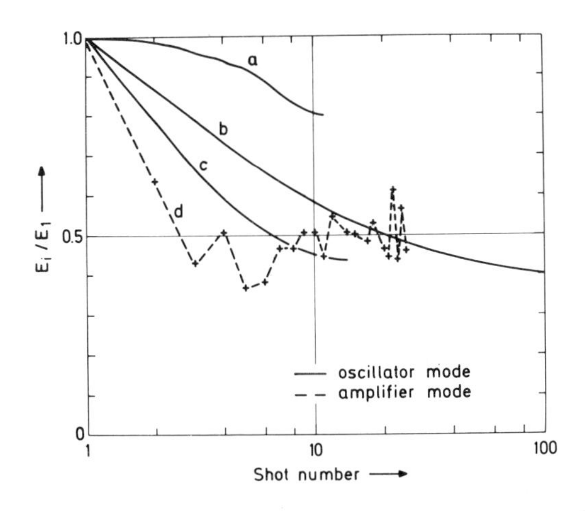

Fig. 2.8. Laser output energy normalized to the value of the first shot vs shot number (fast flash photolysis). (a) 13 mbar i-C_3F_7I [2.84], (b) 40 mbar i-C_3F_7I + 100 mbar SF_6 [2.90], (c) 67 mbar i-C_3F_7I [2.84], (d) 85 mbar i-C_3F_7I + 700 mbar SF_6 [2.91]

relatively important parameters: the amount of pumping energy deposited in the laser medium, the parent gas pressure, the time interval between successive shots (which determines the diffusion rate of I_2 out of the active zone), the volume ratio of the active and the passive zone of the laser tube (which affects the I_2 dilution in the active zone), and the duration of the pumping process. With respect to the latter point it has been found [2.84] that in the case of *slow* flash photolysis the existence of a quasi-equilibrium state could not be detected; usually after ten shots the laser output had decayed to zero.

In view of such a complex situation it is impossible to predict theoretically what the output energy of a laser will be in an individual experiment when the quasi-equilibrium state is reached. The following discussion is therefore restricted to explaining why a quasi-equilibrium state appears to be possible in principle.

It is assumed that the perfluoroalkyl iodides are suitably pumped or sufficiently diluted that all the effects arising from pyrolysis (thermal cracking of the RI molecule with $f \ll 1$) and overheating of the radicals produced in the photodissociation process can be neglected, especially the hot radical reaction considered by several authors [2.92-98]:

$$R + RI \rightarrow R_2 + I^* . \tag{2.22}$$

This reaction has been suggested as a possible explanation of the "late time gain" apparently observed in some laser experiments [2.96,97]. In addition, the exothermic chain decomposition of RI molecules occurring due to the reaction of radicals and iodine atoms with the parent molecule itself and described by the overall process [2.85]

$$2\ RI \rightarrow R_2 + I_2 \tag{2.23}$$

will not be taken into account.

When considering the regeneration capability of the perfluoroalkyl iodides one first has to realize that the I_2 concentration in the laser medium caused by too rapid dimerization of the radicals (according to the process $2R \rightarrow R_2$) cannot increase indefinitely from shot to shot when the temperature of the laser medium and the laser tube is kept at a constant value either by direct cooling or by waiting a sufficiently long time interval between two successive shots. In such cases the maximum possible value of the I_2 concentration is prescribed by the laser tube temperature according to the vapour pressure curve, e.g. at 20°C $N_I \cong 1 \times 10^{16}\ cm^{-3}$. Excess molecular iodine will condense at the laser tube wall and diffuse into the non-illuminated zones of the laser tube.

Since I_2 is a strong quencher of excited atomic iodine according to the reaction

$$I^* + I_2 \rightarrow I + I_2 \tag{2.24}$$

with a rate constant value of $k_Q = (4\text{-}8) \times 10^{-11}\ cm^3$/s molecule, [2.99-102], an I_2 concentration as low as $1 \times 10^{16} cm^{-3}$ is sufficient to prevent the laser from exceeding the oscillation threshold when the pump rate is small, as reported for some of the experiments [2.84] in Fig. 2.8. Since such behaviour is not observed, one has to postulate the existence of some mechanism that decomposes I_2 during the pumping period. Two processes appear to be possible. The first is the chemical reaction

$$R + I_2 \rightarrow RI + I \tag{2.25}$$

with a rate constant of $k_{Reg} = 4 \times 10^{-12}\ cm^3$/s molecule for $R = CF_3$ [2.103] (for the larger radicals this value should be the same or slightly less). The second is the photolysis of I_2 described by

$$I_2 + h\nu \rightarrow I + I^{(*)} \tag{2.26}$$

which may involve excited atomic iodine. The dissociating radiation is in the visible, around 500 nm. The absorption cross-section and bandwidth are such [2.104,105] that a short-pulse flashlamp with an electron temperature of ~ 12 000 K can effectively dissociate I_2 vapour at a concentration of ~ 10^{16} cm^{-3} within a few μs. This is comparable to the time scale of the chemical reaction (2.25) for typical radical densities of ~ 10^{17} cm^{-3}.

Processes (2.25,26) have to be more rapid than the radical recombination reaction (dimerization)

$$R + R \rightarrow R_2 \tag{2.27}$$

in order to make the regeneration of the laser medium possible. In the case of reaction (2.25) it is direct competition; this reaction is predominant when the ratio $(N_R \cdot k_D)/(N_I \cdot k_{Reg})$ is small relative to unity. When the quasi-equilibrium situation is approached, N_R and N_I are of equal orders of magnitude, so that the ratio k_D/k_{Reg} is only then important and should be as small as possible. According to Table 2.5 this holds for i-C_3F_7I and even more so for t-C_4F_9I.

The photolytic decomposition of I_2 contributes indirectly to the regeneration of the laser medium by producing ground-state iodine atoms which can then recombine with the radicals to form parent molecules according to the reaction

$$R + I \rightarrow RI \ , \tag{2.28}$$

which is very fast (see "k_R" in Table 2.5).

It is clear that reactions (2.25,26) can only be effective when the I_2 concentration has reached a certain value. A rough estimate shows that self-regeneration is initiated at I_2 concentrations of the order of 10^{16} cm^{-3}, i.e. a quasi-equilibrium situation becomes possible. This occurs at the cost of the inversion since the excited iodine atoms are strongly quenched by the I_2 molecules and ground-state iodine atoms are formed by processes (2.25,26). As a consequence, the energy output of an oscillator or amplifier is lowered, the extent depending strongly on the perfluoroalkyl iodide chosen. Here t-C_4F_9I seems to be the candidate with the lowest reduction, but this has not yet been experimentally confirmed.

The number of shots necessary to reach the quasi-equilibrium situation can be estimated from the I_2 concentration appearing after the first shot. In the case of the oscillator mode it will be some fraction of the threshold value of the inversion. In the absence of I_2 diffusion this fraction should have a value of 0.5, otherwise less. 1×10^{15} cm^{-3} will then be a typical value of the I_2 concentration appearing after the first shot. It will then take about 10 shots before self-regeneration of the laser medium can become effective. In the amplifier mode it proceeds more rapidly since an I_2 concentration of 1×10^{16} cm^{-3} can be easily generated with one shot, as is shown in Fig. 2.8.

In the *oscillator mode* the RI regeneration can be further improved if additional radicals are formed in the reaction volume. This has been shown by the addition of hexafluoroacetone as a photolytic CF_3 source [2.85]:

$$(CF_3)_2CO \rightarrow 2\ CF_3 + CO\ . \tag{2.29}$$

It should be noted that the absorption spectra of hexafluoroacetone and CF_3I do not overlap, so that there is no competition with respect to the pumplight. Since the absorption cross-section of hexafluoroacetone is 20 times smaller than that of CF_3I, a large amount of $(CF_3)_2CO$ is necessary in order to generate an appreciable amount of radicals. Unfortunately, $(CF_3)_2CO$ is a strong quencher for excited iodine so that its pressure is limited to several hundred millibars. But even with this restriction a quasi-constant energy output behaviour could be demonstrated for 200 shots, the decrease with respect to the first shot being about 20% [2.85]. This result makes CF_3I together with $(CF_3)_2CO$ an interesting candidate for multiple-shot operation.

For $i\text{-}C_3F_7I$ a radical source with similar absorption and quenching properties also exists: $(C_3F_7)_2CO$. The improvement is not as pronounced as in the case of CF_3I, since $i\text{-}C_3F_7I$ has a much better regeneration capability than CF_3I owing to the longer lifetime of its radicals. The addition of $(C_3F_7)_2CO$ should help to improve the multiple-shot performance; the extent can only be estimated since experimental data are not available at present. But a decrease in the output after several hundred shots which is not larger than 10% relative to the first shot should be within reach.

In summary, at least in the case of $i\text{-}C_3F_7I$, conditions are possible where the dissociation can be balanced by recombination processes without additional radical sources so that starting with a certain shot number the medium consumption becomes negligible. The inversion available in this quasi-equilibrium situation is, however, lower than the one occurring in the first shots. A similar, but somewhat more favourable behaviour, especially with respect to the inversion loss, can be expected from $t\text{-}C_4F_9I$.

The data obtained so far are insufficient to clarify the details and the efficiency of the regeneration process, especially at high repetition rates and shot numbers in excess of 10^3. Only further investigations can answer these questions.

2.3.4 Kinetic Modeling Studies

Kinetic modeling studies of the iodine laser have been reported since 1966 by a large number of authors [2.100,106-119]. During this period of 14 years, increasing agreement regarding the number of reactions considered essential for the kinetics of photodissociated perfluoroalkyl iodides and the value of the pertaining rate constants was achieved. The model accepted at present utilizes the assumption that the photolysis of the alkyl iodides does not lead to the production of hot radicals and thermal decomposition of RI molecules (pyrolysis[2]). It consists of the following processes:

Photodissociation of RI and I_2

1) $RI + h\nu_1 \xrightarrow{0.27\ \mu m} R + fI^* + (1 - f)I$,

2) $I_2 + h\nu_2 \xrightarrow{0.5\ \mu m} 2I$ or $I + I^*$ (see Sect.2.3.3),

Laser action

3) $I^* + h\nu_3 \xrightarrow{1.32\ \mu m} I + 2h\nu_3$,

Collisional deactivation of I^*

4) $I^* + M \rightarrow I + M$($M$ = RI, He, Ne, Ar, Kr, Xe, N_2, CO_2, SF_6, O_2, I_2),

RI regeneration

5) $R + I \rightarrow RI$,

6) $R + I_2 \rightarrow RI + I$,

R dimerization

7) $R + R \rightarrow R_2$,

I_2 formation

8) $2I + M \rightarrow I_2 + M$.

---

[2]Pyrolysis which impairs the laser performance can always be avoided by a suitable amount of buffer gas.

With respect to the radicals, both the recombination process $R^* + I \rightarrow RI$ and the quenching process $I^* + R \rightarrow I + R$ have been omitted. According to [2.100], these two processes are completely inefficient and can be neglected because of the much faster dimerization process $2R \rightarrow R_2$. This statement holds for $R = CF_3$ and $R = {}^{i-}_{n-}\}C_3F_7$; for $R = t\text{-}C_4F_9$, the situation might be different.

The formation of molecular I_2 also needs some comment. Reaction 8 may, in principle, involve one or two excited iodine atoms, for example,

$$I^* + I + RI \rightarrow I_2 + RI \ ,$$
$$I^* + I^* + RI \rightarrow I_2 + RI \ .$$

From energy considerations inferred from the I_2 potential energy curves [2.110,114,115], it can be argued that these recombination reactions should have much smaller rate constants than the reaction involving only ground-state iodine atoms. This conclusion has been experimentally confirmed [2.120], so that reactions involving I^* atoms can indeed be neglected. The same also holds for reactions when the third body is either M or I_2.

The eight processes listed above do not include diffusion effects since their time scales are of the order of seconds compared to the micro- to millisecond time scales of the chemical reactions. For the same reason, spontaneous emission has also been neglected. In the case of single-shot operation (always with a fresh filling of the laser tube), induced emission (process 3) needs only be taken into account for the oscillator mode. For multiple-shot operation using the same gas fill, induced emission is also important for the amplifier mode.

The mathematical formulation of the kinetic rate equations is straightforward and will not be given here. The interested reader is refered to the literature, e.g. [2.117]. The rate data given in Table 2.5 are quasi--room-temperature values (300 K) since the temperature rise of the laser medium caused by the photolysis of the perfluoroalkyl iodides is assumed to be so small that it does not affect the value of the rate constants. This situation usually prevails in the amplifier mode since an appreciable amount of buffer gas is always necessary for energy storage. For the oscillator mode things may be different when the medium is strongly pumped without any buffer gas being present. In such a case the temperature dependence of the rate constants has to be taken into account; moreover, it has to be determined whether pyrolysis can become effective.

The references given in Table 2.5 are the most recent. Where possible, those which critically review previous papers dealing with a similar subject are cited.

Comparisons of computational studies based on the model outlined above with experimental observations have not yet been carried out. Despite this lack of information, the model proposed should be capable of making quantitative predictions accurate to within a factor of 2 with respect to the long-time behaviour of the inversion in an amplifier, the power and energy output of an oscillator as well as the build-up period and final amount of molecular iodine when the excitation conditions are clearly known. Moreover, it should also be applicable to multiple-shot operation; i.e. it should give a qualitatively correct description of the laser performance after many shots without medium replacement.

What has been formulated here as an expectation had apparently already been achieved in some earlier papers where good agreement between the predictions of the model assumed and experimental data is claimed. Such agreements may be artificially generated by fitting the model to the measurements, using the rate constants as adjustable parameters, or by mutual compensation of errors arising from incorrectly chosen values of two or more rate constants.

More accurate predictions can be obtained from the model proposed here when additional complexities of the iodine laser system are taken into account, such as magnetic field effects, shock waves and acoustic waves (see Sect. 4.2). The latter arise from inhomogeneous heating of the laser medium [2.100,131-133] and introduce optical inhomogeneities similar to those due to the shock waves.

For the case of short-flash photolysis with pumping times not exceeding 10 μs and single-shot operation, the kinetic model becomes much simpler since collisional deactivation of I^* and all the processes involving molecular iodine can then be neglected, leading to the reduced set of processes

1) $RI + h\nu_1 \xrightarrow{0.27\ \mu m} R + fI^* + (1 - f)I$,

3) $I^* + h\nu_3 \xrightarrow{1.32\ \mu m} I + 2\ h\nu_3$,

5) $R + I \rightarrow RI$,

7) $R + R \rightarrow R_2$.

When attention is further restricted to the amplifier mode, the inversion is simply some fraction of the time integral of the pump rate when f is close to unity [2.89].

Table 2.5. Rate constants for quenching of I^*, recombination, dimerization, formation of molecular iodine and regeneration

n=1 bi-molecular reaction, n=2 ter-molecular reaction

Reaction	n	Molecule	Rate constant $\left[\frac{cm^{3n}}{molecule^n s}\right]$	Ref
$I^* + RI \rightarrow I + RI$	1	RI =		
		CF_3I	2×10^{-17}	2.121
			$(3.3\pm0.5)\times10^{-17}$	2.122
		C_2F_5I	$(1.8\pm0.1)\times10^{-17}$	2.5
			$(2.1\pm0.2)\times10^{-17}$	2.122
		$n\text{-}C_3F_7I$	$(4.6\pm0.3)\times10^{-17}$	2.123
			$(1.7\pm0.2)\times10^{-17}$	2.122
		$i\text{-}C_3F_7I$	$(2.0\pm0.2)\times10^{-17}$	2.122
		$t\text{-}C_4F_9I$	$(7\pm2)\times10^{-16}$	2.124
$I^* + M \rightarrow I + M$	1	M =		
		He, Ne, Ar, Kr, Xe	$<2\times10^{-18}$	2.125
		N_2	5.2×10^{-17}	2.126
				2.125
		CO_2	1.5×10^{-16}	2.125
			4.6×10^{-16}	2.16
		SF_6	2.4×10^{-17}	2.125
		O_2	2.5×10^{-11}	2.126
		I_2	3.0×10^{-11}	2.101
			8.0×10^{-11}	2.100
			3.6×10^{-11}	2.102
$R + I \rightarrow RI$	1	R =		
		CF_3	$(1.6\pm0.3)\times10^{-11}$	2.86
			$(0.9\pm1.6)\times10^{-11}$	2.127
		$n\text{-}C_3F_7$	$(0.8\pm0.4)\times10^{-11}$	2.86
			$(0.7\pm0.1)\times10^{-11}$	2.127
		$i\text{-}C_3F_7$	$(1.0\pm0.4)\times10^{-11}$	2.127
		$t\text{-}C_4F_9$	$(0.6\pm0.1)\times10^{-11}$	2.86

Reaction	n	Molecule	Rate constant $\left[\frac{cm^{3n}}{molecule^n s}\right]$	Ref.
$R + R \rightarrow R_2$	1	R =		
		CF_3	$(5.5\pm1.2)\times10^{-12}$	2.86
			$(5.5\pm0.7)\times10^{-12}$	2.127
		$n\text{-}C_3F_7$	$(3\pm1.3)\times10^{-12}$	2.86
			$(2\pm0.3)\times10^{-12}$	2.127
		$i\text{-}C_3F_7$	$(0.65\pm0.1)\times10^{-12}$	2.127
		$t\text{-}C_4F_9$	$<0.2\times10^{-12}$	2.86
			3×10^{-14} a)	2.119
$2I + M \rightarrow I_2 + M$	2	M =		
		He	2.8×10^{-33}	2.128
		Ne	3.7×10^{-33}	2.128
		Ar	6.5×10^{-33}	2.129
		Kr	1.2×10^{-32}	2.128
		Xe	1.5×10^{-32}	2.128
		N_2	2.3×10^{-32}	2.130
		CO_2	6.9×10^{-32}	2.130
		SF_6	6×10^{-32} b)	2.100
		CF_3I	1.3×10^{-31}	2.100
			1.5×10^{-31}	2.115
		C_3F_7I	4.5×10^{-31}	2.115
			3.8×10^{-31}	2.116
		I_2	2.9×10^{-30}	2.115
			3.7×10^{-30}	2.129
$R + I_2 \rightarrow RI + I$	1	R =		
		CF_3	4.0×10^{-12}	2.103

a) Extrapolated from the values of the smaller radicals

b) Rough estimate

*2.3.5 Inversion Losses by Quenching of I**

When a constant pump rate is assumed, the relative inversion loss due to quenching of I* is found to be (ground state originally not populated, f=1)

$$\frac{\Delta N_{ideal} - \Delta N}{\Delta N_{ideal}} \simeq \frac{2}{3}\frac{T_p}{t_Q} \tag{2.30}$$

where ΔN_{ideal} is the inversion without quenching and t_Q the characteristic time scale of the quenching process given by

$$1/t_Q = N_{RI}k_{RI} + N_{BG}k_{BG} + N_{O_2}k_{O_2} + N_{J_2}k_{J_2} \quad . \tag{2.31}$$

Here N_i denotes the number density of the species i, and k_i the pertinent rate constant (see Table 2.5). In (2.30) it has been further assumed that $T_p \lesssim 0.4\ t_Q$ holds.

According to (2.31) the quenching agents are RI molecules, the buffer gas and molecular iodine. Oxygen is not harmful as long as its concentration is far below that of the excited iodine atoms. This is due to the fact that the quenching rate constants for $O_2(^1\Delta)$ (see (2.16)) are small, $\sim 10^{-20}$ cm^3/s molecule for the noble gases and $\sim 10^{-18}$ cm^3/s molecule for CO_2, SF_6 and the alkyl iodides [2.134]. The lifetime of the O_2 $(^1\Delta)$ molecules is thus of the order of milliseconds or larger for typical amplifier conditions. Since the pump duration is much shorter than one millisecond, only a small fraction of the excited iodine atoms can be deactivated by the oxygen molecules.

The condition $N_{O_2} \ll N_{I^*}$ is usually met when research grade gases with an oxygen inpurity level of 2 ppm are used. For a buffer gas pressure of 4 bar the oxygen number density amounts then to $\sim 2 \times 10^{14}$ cm^{-3} which is small compared to 10^{16}-10^{17} cm^{-3} which is the typical range for I* number densities. This means that the inversion loss due to oxygen quenching is not larger than 1% and can therefore be neglected.

More serious is the influence of molecular iodine on the inversion, especially when a regeneration system is employed [2.90]. In this case the I_2 concentration is controlled by the temperature of the cold trap and lies in the range from 10^{13} to 10^{14} cm^{-3}. Similar values should also be encountered in amplifiers using a fresh filling for each shot. After each firing a certain amount of I_2 remains in the laser tube so that the I_2 concentration increases from shot to shot until an equilibrium value is reached. The build-up of an appreciable I_2 concentration can be avoided when the laser tube is evacuated down to 10^{-6} mbar between two shots. However, this requires expensive pumps and long evacuation times so that it is not a solution which is practically feasible. Another I_2 source is the alkyl iodide itself. Both contributions result in an I_2 concentration lying in the region given above.

Table 2.6 presents some t_Q values for a laser medium with either argon, SF_6 or CO_2 as the buffer gas at three different pressures, 1,3 and 5 bar. It turned out that the contribution of the RI molecules to t_Q is negligible because of their low partial pressure ($\leqq$ 30 mbar assumed). The figures for $N_{I_2} = 1 \times 10^{12}$ cm^{-3} are almost equal to those valid for a laser medium free of any I_2. This is, however, difficult to realize, especially under the condition of a large size, high-energy storage amplifier fired each 10 minutes. If a realistic N_{I_2} value of about 3×10^{13} cm^{-3} is adopted and the condition of a small inversion loss of $\leqq$ 10% is to be met (see (2.30)), the maximum allowable pump duration becomes 100 μs for argon. This value is independent of pressure. For SF_6 and CO_2 a strong pressure dependance occurs. If a pumping time not longer than 20 μs is assumed - this value arises from the need to avoid gasdynamic perturbations (see Chap. 4) - than SF_6 can be used up to pressures of 8 bar and CO_2 up to pressures of 2 bar. A lower pressure limit arises for SF_6 when a regeneration system is employed. This is due to the fact that SF_6 condenses below -30°C at pressures above 3 bar.

Table 2.6. Quenching time t_Q for a laser medium with either argon, SF_6 or CO_2 as the buffer gas at five different I_2 concentrations. Values of the quenching rate constants used (in cm^3/s molecule): argon 2×10^{-19}, SF_6 2.4×10^{-17}, CO_2 1.5×10^{-16}, I_2 3×10^{-11}, RI 2×10^{-17}

N_{I_2} [cm^{-3}]	$t_{Ar,Q}$[μs]			$t_{SF_6,Q}$[μs]			$t_{CO_2,Q}$[μs]		
	1 bar	3 bar	5bar	1 bar	3 bar	5 bar	1 bar	3 bar	5 bar
1×10^{15}	33	33	33	33	32	30	30	25	21
1×10^{14}	332	331	330	279	211	170	151	72	48
3×10^{13}	1087	1075	1064	671	378	264	222	85	53
1×10^{13}	3125	3030	2941	1122	489	313	255	90	55
1×10^{12}	20000	16700	14290	1610	564	342	274	92	55

Since the broadening coefficients of SF_6 and argon are equal, argon is the better perfoming buffer gas. This statement only holds with the respect to the quenching behaviour. If gasdynamic and heat capacity aspects are predominant, the situation is reversed (see Chap. 4).

With regard to energy storage CO_2 is attractive because of its broadening coefficient which is twice as large as that of argon. Although the pressure of CO_2 is limited to 2 bar it can still be used to minimize the pressure necessary to realize a prescribed value of the medium linewidth; f.e., when this value amounts to 23 GHz enabling a stored energy density of $\sim 8\ J/cm^2$, an argon pressure of 6 bar is required. The same linewidth can also be obtained with a mixture of 2 bar CO_2 and 2 bar argon. The pressure reduction is thus 2 bar and lowers the mechanical loading of the laser tube and windows considerably, especially for large diameters. This solution is, however, only feasible when the pumping time is sufficiently short, i.e. smaller than 20 μs.

3. Principles of High-Power Operation

High-power operation of an iodine laser involves the generation of a short pulse and subsequent amplification of this pulse in a chain of amplifiers. Physical and technical aspects of such an arrangement are reviewed in this chapter.

The first section deals with various methods for short pulse generation. The emphasis is on active mode locking since this is the most widely used technique, but a number of alternatives are also discussed.

In the second section the basic laws governing the energy storage properties of an amplifier as determined by technical and physical constraints are derived. Equations relating the minimum length and diameter of an amplifier to the desired energy of the output pulse are given.

The last section treats the theory of pulse propagation in iodine laser amplifiers. First the basic equations for coherent and incoherent pulse propagation in homogeneously broadened media are reviewed. Next, the complications arising from the hyperfine structure of the iodine laser transition are discussed. Approximations used to deal with this special feature are described. Finally coherent pulse propagation in iodine laser amplifiers is treated in detail including predictions from a computer code with regard to pulse distortion and energy extraction in a laser amplifier chain.

3.1 Short-Pulse Generation

The techniques used for generating short iodine laser pulses are similar to the ones applied to other laser materials, such as ruby or Nd glass. The methods mainly employed are Q switching, pulse cutting and active mode locking. Two further methods which have been proven to be suitable in principle are passive mode locking and free induction decay.

3.1.1 Q Switching and Gain Switching

Q-switched as well as gain-switched operation provide laser pulses with similar time behaviour. Both techniques are based on the same working principle: the gain is raised far above the threshold value, thereby permitting the laser to emit a single "giant" pulse.

The two methods differ, however, in the way the inversion is raised well above its threshold value. The Q-switch method is based on keeping the resonator losses high until the inversion achieves a high value. Then the resonator quality (or "Q") is suddenly switched to its maximum possible value. In gain switching the laser is pumped much faster than the buildup time of the pulse, resulting in high excess inversion.

Q switching in iodine lasers has been achieved by the use of rotating prisms [3.1], by modulation of magnetic fields [3.2,3] and by shock waves [3.4,5]. These methods are useful in oscillator arrangements employing relatively slow flashlamp current circuits (discharge time ~100 μs). Due to gasdynamic disturbances, however, the beam quality of the pulses is usually not adequate for use in experiments requiring low-divergence beams.

Gain switching is simpler and provides a better beam quality than Q switching. The only requirement is a fast flashlamp driving circuit with a discharge time (first current zero) comparable to the pulse buildup time, which is typically about 30-50 cavity round trip times. For a 2.50-m-long cavity, the discharge time should thus be not larger than 1 μs. Under this condition a giant pulse of 50- to 100-ns duration is emitted by the laser. Powers on the order of a MW are easily achieved. Usually the pulse exhibits self mode locking with a temporal structure varying from shot to shot. The peak power, therefore also fluctuates by about a factor of two.

Gain switching has been applied to a recently developed iodine laser oscillator capable of emitting temporally smooth pulses of variable pulse duration [3.6]. The device is based on using an excimer laser as the optical pumping source. The excimer laser can be either a KrF laser (λ = 248 nm) or a XeCl laser (λ = 308 nm), and the radiation can be applied transversally or longitudinally to the laser axis.

If the 10 to 20 ns pulse duration of the pump laser is shorter than the buildup time of the pulse, the dynamics of the gain-switched pulse are decoupled from the pumping process. Within certain limits the pulse duration can therefore be varied simply by changing the cavity length. To avoid temporal substructure caused by beating of axial modes, the gain bandwidth should allow only one axial mode to oscillate. This is achieved by matching the iodide pressure and therefore the pressure broadening linewidth of the medium to the cavity length. Single transverse mode operation is enforced by an appropriate mode iris in the cavity.

With excimer laser pumping energies of a few hundred mJ, the iodine laser emits smooth, diffraction-limited pulses in the mJ range. Pulses with durations variable between 2 and 12 ns are obtained. Experimental parameters for three cavity lengths are summarized in Table 3.1.

An extension of the range of pulse durations is possible down to about 0.5 ns, limited by a practical minimum cavity length and by the requirement that the pump pulse be terminated before the emission of the iodine laser pulse. The upper limit for the generation of smooth pulses is determined by the Doppler width of the laser transition and is expected to be around 30 ns.

Table 3.1. Experimental parameters of an excimer laser pumped oscillator for three cavity lengths. Excimer laser pumping energy 500 mJ. Reflectivity of output coupler 34%

Cavity length [cm]	i-C_3F_7I pressure[mbar]	Delay time[ns]	Pulse duration[ns]	Pulse energy[mJ]
10	370	32	2.6	1.4
20	200	40	4.8	0.95
40	67	90	12.0	0.28

3.1.2 Pulse Cutting

A very flexible method of obtaining a pulse with a duration from subnanosecond to several tens of nanoseconds is to "cut" the pulse electrooptically from a much longer laser pulse. Kerr cells [3.7] and Pockels cells [3.8] can be used as a switch. Pulses as short as 300 ps can be realized with this method.

To obtain a reproducible pulse with an approximately rectangular pulse shape it is necessary to have a master oscillator with a smooth temporal profile, devoid of self mode locking. To achieve this, the oscillator has to run on a single axial mode. This can be obtained with a short cavity length and low iodide pressure with no buffer gas. In this case the energy of the master pulses is quite small and further amplification is necessary to drive a laser triggered spark gap.

Nevertheless, pulse cutting provides a useful method for generating short pulses, the main advantage being the ease of varying the pulse length over a range of about two orders of magnitude.

3.1.3 Active Mode Locking

This is the most widely used method for generating short iodine laser pulses. In active mode locking a modulator close to one of the mirrors modulates the circulating radiation with a frequency corresponding to the inverse of the cavity roundtrip time. The oscillator is thus forced to oscillate in such a way that a short pulse (shorter than the cavity roundtrip time) travels back and forth in the resonator passing through the modulator at the time of its maximum transmission. The laser then emits a train of pulses separated by the cavity roundtrip time. The modulation frequency $2\,f_m$ of the modulator is approximately $c/2\ell$ where ℓ is the optical path length in the resonator. The duration of the pulses is determined by an equilibrium between the shortening action of the modulator and the lengthening effect of the medium bandwidth. This fact is expressed by the equation for the pulse duration in a homogeneously broadened active medium, first derived by SIEGMAN and co-workers [3.9],

$$\tau_p = \frac{(2\ \ln 2)^{\frac{1}{2}}}{\pi}\,\frac{g_o^{\frac{1}{4}}}{\delta_m^{\frac{1}{2}}}\,\frac{1}{(f_m \Delta\nu_p)^{\frac{1}{2}}}\ , \tag{3.1}$$

which is valid for amplitude modulation. In this equation g_o stands for the dimensionless threshold gain-length product, δ_m for the modulation index, f_m for the driver frequency of the modulator and $\Delta\nu_p$ for the pressure--broadened linewidth. The modulation index is defined by the single pass amplitude transmission function of the modulator

$$a(t) = \cos[\delta_m \sin(2\pi f_m t)]\ . \tag{3.2}$$

Usual values of δ_m range from 1.0 to 1.6, corresponding to an intensity modulation from 70% to almost 100%.

The expression $g_o^{1/4}/\delta_m^{1/2}$ is usually close to unity so that (3.1) can be approximated by

$$\tau_p = 0.37/(f_m \Delta\nu_p)^{\frac{1}{2}} \quad . \tag{3.3}$$

Medium bandwidth limited pulses ($\tau_p \cong 1/\Delta\nu_p$) can thus only be achieved when $\Delta\nu_p/f_m \cong 10$ holds. This can be realized in short cavities of about 1-m length at medium linewidths $\Delta\nu_p \cong 1$ GHz. Therefore only ns pulses can become bandwidth limited; for shorter pulses the inverse bandwidth $1/\Delta\nu_p$ will always be much smaller than the pulse width.

In pulsed lasers it has to be ascertained that the equilibrium pulse duration given by (3.1) is reached during the buildup of the pulse. The number m of roundtrips necessary for steady state is given by [3.10]

$$m > \frac{0.38\Delta\nu_p}{\sqrt{g_m}\delta_m f_m} \tag{3.4}$$

where g_m is the dimensionless gain-length product during pulse buildup.

Turning now to the experimental situation in iodine lasers, we note that in most cases an acousto-optic mode locker is used [3.11-13]. Electro--optic mode locking is applied less frequently [3.14,15] owing to the problems of combined high-frequency and high-voltage electronics. An acousto-optic mode locker consists of a transducer, usually an x-cut quartz platelet, driving a rectangular block of a suitable acousto-optic material, e.g. fused silica. A convenient driving frequency is 30 MHz, and since the modulation frequency is twice the driving frequency of the transducer, the corresponding resonator length is $\ell = 2.50$ m. It should be noted that due to gain-induced dispersion the length of the resonator is effectively reduced: In a gain medium the group velocity v_g of a laser pulse is somewhat smaller than the speed of light, owing to the anomalous dispersion of an inverted line. For a Lorentzian lineshape the following equation holds

$$v_g = \frac{c}{n_o + \frac{cg_c}{2\pi\Delta\nu_p}} \tag{3.5}$$

where n_o stands for the normal refractive index of the buffer gas, g_c for the gain at line centre and $\Delta\nu_p$ for the FWHM of the Lorentzian laser line [3.16]. Under ordinary conditions, the shortening of the cavity length amounts typically to only 0.3-3 cm in an iodine oscillator.

If the length of the resonator is well matched to the modulator frequency, at an intensity modulation depth of 70-80% a pulse train such as that shown in Fig. 3.1 is emitted by an iodine laser. The envelope of the pulse train is determined by the saturation of the gain by the pulse travelling back and forth in the cavity. The dependence of the pulse duration on the argon buffer gas pressure is shown in Fig. 3.2. The experimental points are in good agreement with the theoretical curve, [see (3.1)]. This agreement indicates that the pulse shape has attained its asymptotic value. The shortest pulses generated by the active mode locking of an iodine laser had a duration of 160 ps and were obtained at an argon buffer gas pressure of 7.9 bar [3.17].

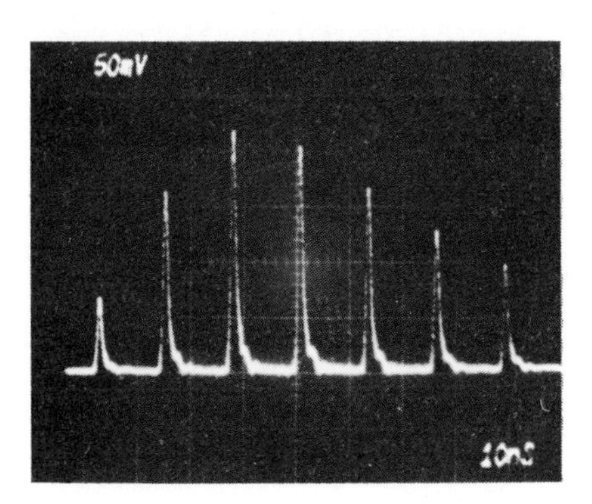

Fig. 3.1. Pulse train emitted by an actively mode-locked iodine laser

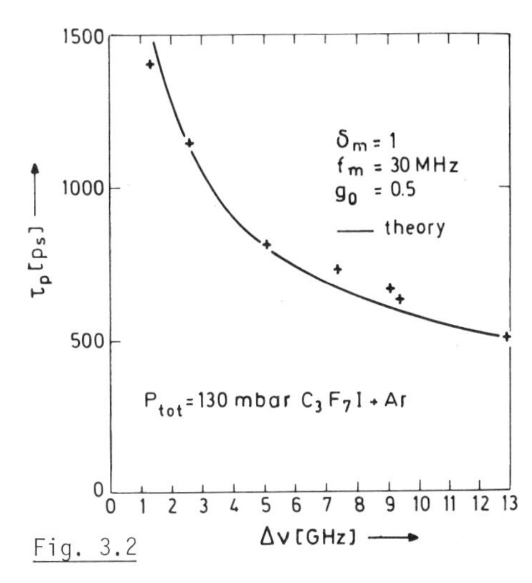

Fig. 3.2

Fig. 3.2. Pulselengths of an actively mode-locked iodine laser as a function of the pressure of the active medium. Comparison of experimental values (+ + +) with Siegman-Kuizenga theory

3.1.4 Passive Mode Locking

In passive mode locking a saturable absorber is placed within the laser vavity close to one of the mirrors. The effect of the absorber is to single out the strongest laser pulse from the fluorescent noise which is subsequently amplified until it bleaches the dye. After the passive Q switch opens, the dynamics are similar to the case of active mode locking. Passive mode locking is not as reliable as active mode locking since the process is basically a statistical one.

Passive mode locking has been relatively little explored with iodine lasers. There is actually only one report on successful operation of a passively mode locked laser [3.18]. The main reason is that useful saturable absorbers at 1315 nm have become available only recently.

Narrow bandwidth saturable absorbers used for prepulse suppression in iodine laser chains [3.19] cannot be applied to passive mode locking since the laser would "bypass" the absorber by oscillating in the wings of the gain line.

Wide bandwidth dye saturable absorbers for the iodine laser have been developed during the last years. The dithiene BDN II was proposed as a saturable absorber at 1.3 μm by DREXHAGE and REYNOLDS [3.20]. Passive mode locking of an iodine laser was demonstrated using BDN II dissolved in dimethylsulphoxide [3.18]. Complete bleaching of BDN II is impossible however, due to the four-level structure and strong excited-state absorption [3.21]. A group at the Lebedev Institute has developed a saturable absorber with somewhat better saturation behaviour at 1.3 μm [3.22], but passive mode locking was not reported.

A more recently developed dithiene, Jul 2 [3.23], exhibits strongly improved properties compared with BDN II: The molar absorption coefficient (ε = 50000 l mol^{-1}cm^{-1}) is a factor of 1.5 larger and the wavelength of the absorption maximum is around 1.3 μm in numerous neutral solvents. The dye has been used for the decoupling of amplifiers [3.24] but passive mode locking has not yet been attempted.

3.1.5 Free Induction Decay

Free induction decay (FID) was first employed by YABLONOVITCH and GOLDHAR [3.25] to obtain subnanosecond CO_2 laser pulses. The principle is as follows: A long pulse is truncated by a fast switch and passes through an absorber operated in the small-signal regime. The absorber strongly attenuates the initial portion of the pulse. But at the point where the pulse is truncated, the polarization induced in the absorber cannot follow the fast truncation and locally decays with the dephasing time. A local FID pulse of about the same length as the dephasing time is generated and is shortened even more by propagation effects.

Applying this technique to the iodine laser a 2.5-ns pulse from an iodine oscillator was truncated by gas breakdown in a nitrogen cell and then passed through a hot I_2 absorber operated in the small-signal regime.

Streak camera studies of such pulses showed that the breakdown time was about 40 ps and the FID pulse had a FWHM of 100 to 200 ps [3.26, 27].

3.2 Scaling Laws and Energy Storage Capabilities of Iodine Laser Amplifiers

The classical concept of high-power storage lasers involves generation of a short pulse in an oscillator and subsequent amplification in a series of amplifiers. The preamplifiers are operated more or less in the small-signal regime, whereas the large aperture amplifiers, which contribute the main part of the energy, are operated in the saturation regime.

Despite its high space requirements and the associated costs, this concept is being used in essentially all existing high-power laser systems. Other concepts are being examined and may eventually be used in very large laser facilities.

In this section the discussion is limited to the above-mentioned classical concept. Scaling laws and limitations for saturated amplifiers will be derived. The principal parameter determining the sizes of energy amplifiers is the desired output energy E_{out} of the laser pulse. The pulse length, which is of the order of a nanosecond or less, then specifies the output power of the system.

The following points have to be considered by the designer:

- damage threshold of the output window,
- capability for storing high-energy densities.
- homogeneity of the inversion profile, and
- ability to pump enough energy into the required volume.

The obvious desire to design an amplifier as compactly as possible to save space and cost is subject to various restrictions imposed on the parameters of an amplifier. In the following, we will discuss in more detail the requirements for achieving the previously mentioned features.

3.2.1 Amplifier Diameter

The most obvious restriction on the laser amplifier aperture arises from the need to avoid optical damage to the output window. An extensive literature on optical damage of bare surfaces and various coatings is available (see for example [3.28]). Since damage thresholds have a statistical distribution from sample to sample, a compromise must be found between the risk of optical damage and the costs associated with the construction of laser amplifiers having large diameters. This compromise results in a design value e_m for the maximum energy loading of the output window, yielding a minimum diameter

$$d_{min} = 2\sqrt{\frac{E_{out}}{\pi e_m}} \tag{3.6}$$

for this window. It is recommended in Sect. 5.3.3 that e_m is limited to being half the median damage threshold.

In the case of an AR-coated window the damage threshold measurements of LOWDERMILK and MILAM [3.29] suggest a maximum energy loading of $e_m = 4\ J/cm^2$ at a pulse duration of 1 ns. Thus for a 1-kJ laser a minimum diameter of 21 cm is obtained from (3.6). On the other hand, with an uncoated output window or a graded index AR surface, considerably higher energy loadings can be tolerated leading to a more compact laser. If the laser is to be designed for variable pulse durations, the dependence of the energy damage threshold on pulse duration has to be taken into account (Sect. 5.3.3).

3.2.2 *Maximum Stored Energy*

An entirely different consideration leads to a quantitative estimate of the maximum energy that can be stored in an amplifier of given diameter, limited by parasitic oscillations. Stored energy in an amplifier is invariably associated with small-signal amplification, as expressed by the basic formulae

$$e_{st} = h\nu\Delta N\ell, \qquad A_{ss} = \exp(\sigma\Delta N\ell) \tag{3.7}$$

where

e_{st} = inversion energy stored per cm^2 of amplifier
ΔN = inversion density
ℓ = length of the amplifier
σ = maximum cross-section for stimulated emission
A_{ss} = small-signal amplification

The maximum small-signal amplification of an amplifier is limited by the onset of parasitic oscillations from feedback somewhere in the system. This feedback may be caused by reflections from external structures, by dust particles on the windows or by spiralling parasitic modes in the amplifier tube. An empirical upper limit for stable operation of an amplifier is a small-signal amplification of $A_{ss} = 10^2 - 10^3$. Using $A_{ss} = 10^3$, it is easy to derive from the above formulae the maximum stored energy per cm^2 of amplifier cross-section

$$e_{max} = \frac{h\nu}{\sigma} \ln A_{ss} \approx 7 \frac{h\nu}{\sigma} \quad . \tag{3.8}$$

It should be pointed out that this estimate is only valid for a single amplifier. In an amplifier chain the maximum stable amplification of an amplifier is reduced by the coupling of the amplifiers unless precautions are taken to effectively decouple one amplifier from another.

It follows from (3.8) that the stored energy of an amplifier can be increased by reducing the stimulated emission cross-section. In an iodine laser this can be done by adding a buffer gas to the laser gas mixture to broaden the line. At high enough buffer gas pressures one has $\sigma \sim 1/p$, and the storable energy scales approximately in proportion to the buffer gas pressure. In principle, therefore, with regard to amplifier *instability* the stored energy density in an amplifier can be made arbitrarily high by raising the buffer gas pressure (see Fig. 3.3). However, the problems associated with the handling of gas pressures significantly above 6 bar in large volumes limit the stored energy density to about 6.5 J/cm^2. Assuming a reasonable extraction efficiency of 50%, the output energy density will be 3.5 - 4 J/cm^2.

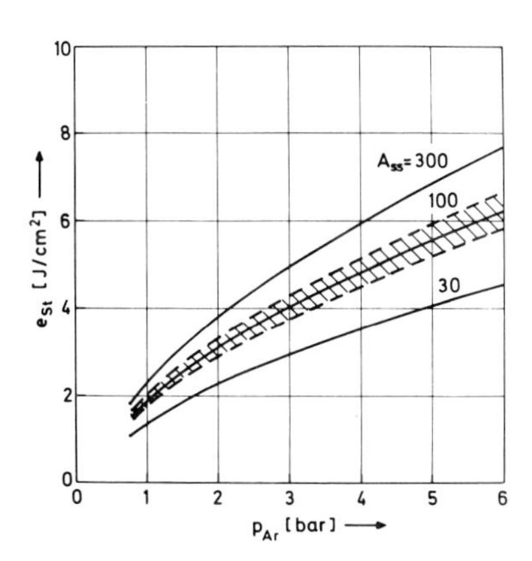

Fig. 3.3. Maximum storable energy density as a function of argon buffer gas pressure with small-signal amplification as a parameter. The iodide pressure is assumed to be negligible ($p_{RI} \leq 20$ mbar). The hatched region around $A_{ss} = 100$ reflects uncertainty in the Einstein A coefficient and pressure broadening coefficient of argon

It should be mentioned that there is another very important reason for adding a buffer gas to the iodide: A minimum amount of buffer gas is needed to prevent the gas from reaching a temperature above 1000°C, which would lead to pyrolysis (see Sect. 2.3). However, even under strong pumping conditions, an argon pressure of less than 1 bar is usually sufficient.

3.2.3 Optimum Iodide Pressure

A condition for the maximum iodide pressure and for the minimum length of an amplifier results from the need to design an optically pumped amplifier with a transverse inversion profile as homogeneous as possible. In the usual pumping arrangements the laser gas in the tube is excited by external flashlamps. Because of the absorption of the pump light by the iodide, an inversion profile with a minimum at the centre of the tube is established. To make the inversion profile as homogeneous as possible, the pressure of the iodide has to be matched to the diameter of the tube. An optimum pressure exists which is high enough to absorb the greater portion of the pumping light but still provides a fairly homogeneous inversion profile. A decrease of 30% in inversion density from the wall to the centre of the tube can usually be tolerated.

The condition for optimum pumping will be approximately fulfilled if the absorption length in the iodide is of the order of the radius of the tube. Under this condition the iodide pressure should be varied in inverse proportion to the tube diameter. The following rule relating the optimum iodide pressure p_{RI} to the tube diameter d has been empirically established [3.30]:

$$p_{RI}d = 200 \text{ mbar cm} \quad . \tag{3.9}$$

This equation serves, of course, only as a general guideline for the choice of the iodide pressure in an amplifier. In practice the pressure required for a particular design depends on the pumping geometry and the amount of inversion inhomogeneity that can be tolerated in a system.

The requirement of a homogeneous inversion profile has a decisive influence on the inversion energy which can be pumped into a given volume. The pumping energy absorbed per cubic centimetre is proportional to the iodide pressure. The need to reduce the iodide pressure with increasing diameter will lead to reduced energy content per unit volume.

If the iodide pressure is scaled according to (3.9) and the flux of pumping light entering the laser tube is assumed to be constant, the energy per unit volume scales inversely to the tube diameter. If an amplifier is to be scaled with a stored energy density complying with the limits derived previously, the length of the amplifier has to be increased in proportion to its diameter.

To determine approximately the dimensions of an amplifier with a given energy content the specific inversion energy density u in millijoule per mbar RI pressure and cubic centimetre is a useful quantity. It has been established experimentally that u is of the order of 1 $mJ/mbar\ cm^3$ in a well-designed amplifier, corresponding to about 20% dissociation. From this latter value it also becomes clear that bleaching of the medium by the pumping light plays only a minor role in iodine laser amplifiers.

A point which should not be overlooked when designing an iodine laser amplifier is the fact that the useful diameter for pulse propagation is decreased by shock waves travelling from the walls of the laser tube towards the centre. In the region of the shock wave, the transmitted wave front of the laser pulse is severely distorted. These shock waves travel slightly faster than the velocity of sound which for a gas consisting mainly of argon means that about 8 mm of the tube diameter is lost for 10 μs of pumping time. For pulse propagation calculations, therefore, instead of the geometrical diameter d of the tube, an effective diameter

$$d_{eff} = d - 2\,T_p a_s - \varphi \ell \tag{3.10}$$

has to be used, where T_p is the pumping time, a_s the velocity of the shock wave, φ the beam divergence (full angle, in general $\leqq 1$ mrad), and ℓ the length of the amplifier (3.13).

3.2.4 Scaling Laws

The considerations discussed in this section (3.6,8,9) may be summarized in the following scaling laws for the diameter d_{eff}, length ℓ and iodide pressure p_{RI} with regard to the desired output energy E_{out} of a fluence-limited amplifier:

$$d_{eff} \sim E_{out}^{1/2} \quad , \quad \ell \sim d_{eff} \sim E_{out}^{1/2} \quad , \quad p_{RI} \sim E_{out}^{-1/2} \ . \tag{3.11}$$

Explicit formulae can be derived by using

$$E_{out} = \frac{\pi d_{eff}^2}{4} \ell u \, p_{RI} \eta_{ex} \qquad (3.12)$$

where η_{ex} is extraction efficiency of the laser pulse. Its value is approximately 0.5 in a well-designed amplifier chain. Equation 3.12 is only approximately valid since the input energy has been neglected in this expression.

Together with (3.6) and (3.9) one obtains

$$d_{eff} = 2\sqrt{\frac{E_{out}}{\pi e_m}} \quad , \quad \ell = \frac{10}{u \eta_{ex}} \sqrt{\frac{E_{out}\, e_m}{\pi}} \quad , \quad p_{RI} = 100\sqrt{\frac{\pi e_m}{E_{out}}} \qquad (3.13)$$

where all the symbols have been defined previously. The above formulae and scaling laws should only be used to give a first-order estimate of the dimensions required for an amplifier. In any real system special requirements or special solutions may lead to considerable deviations from these first-order parameters.

For example, a different pumping geometry might alter the considerations leading to an optimum iodide pressure. A pumping arrangement in which the flashlamps are imaged into the laser tube by some focusing optics might allow a higher pressure than that given by eq. (3.9) to obtain a homogeneous inversion profile.

The scaling laws given by (3.11) can also be circumvented by placing the flashlamps inside the laser medium. Such a design has been reported in [3.31]. In this amplifier the flashlamps are placed in several layers in the active medium, perpendicular to the laser beam. The laser beam is, therefore, split into several sections. The advantage of this configuration is the possibility of extrapolation to larger diameters without any decrease of the stored energy density.

For an experimental demonstration a 38 cm diameter, a 1.7-m long amplifier with 256 flashlamps has been built. A stored energy density of 4 J/liter at a pumping efficiency of 0.6% was obtained. Figure 3.4, adopted from the data of [3.31], shows the dependence of the stored energy density of the "layer amplifier" and of a conventional design with external flashlamps. At diameters larger than 50 cm the design with internal flashlamps exhibits a larger stored energy density than the conventional design.

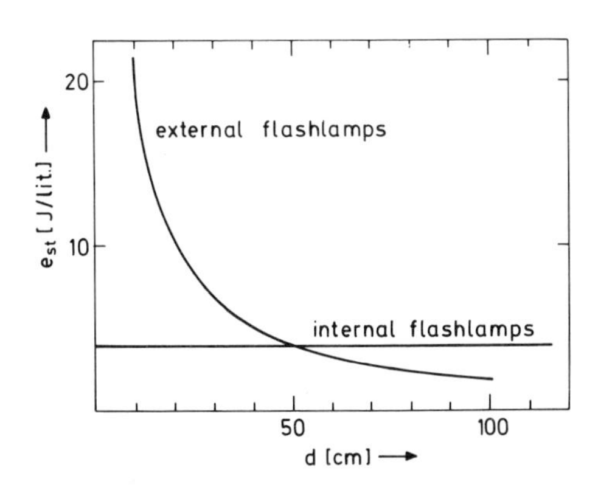

Fig. 3.4. Stored energy density versus beam diameter for conventional design (external flashlamps) and layer amplifier (internal flashlamps)

The scaling laws derived for the main amplifiers do not apply for preamplifiers of an amplifier chain. A preamplifier is usually much less saturated than a main amplifier, and therefore the energy loading of the output window is relatively low. In other words a preamplifier is usually designed with a diameter which is larger than the minimum diameter given by (3.6). The minimum diameter of a preamplifier is essentially determined by the need to propagate the beam through it without being impaired by the shock wave. Guidelines for the outlay of a preamplifier will be given in Sect. 5.1.2.

3.3 Pulse Propagation in Iodine Laser Amplifiers

Pulse propagation in an iodine laser amplifier is characterized by the features of a Lorentzian gain line subject to saturation. Various kinds of pulse distortion result from these two features, depending on the line width of the amplifier, the inversion density and the power of the pulse. For example, pulses with energies far below the saturation density are invariably broadened in an iodine laser amplifier because of the finite bandwidth of the gain medium. On the other hand, strong, saturating pulses may be shortened upon amplification because saturation can have a steepening effect. It depends on the exact parameters, which effect dominates and what the final pulse width is.

An important point arises from the hyperfine spectrum of the iodine laser transition, which has a decisive influence on energy extraction and a less pronounced influence on pulse shaping.

3.3.1 General Considerations

In this section we discuss theories of pulse propagation under these conditions and predictions of energy extraction and pulse distortion. Examples of numerical calculations of pulse shapes under various conditions are given. The treatment will be one dimensional.

A short review of the "coherent" and "incoherent" pulse propagation equations and a discussion of their relevance in iodine laser amplifiers is appropriate.

In a two-level system the propagation of a pulse in x direction with an electric field (in V/m) is given by

$$E(x,t) = \frac{1}{2}\{\mathcal{E}(x,t)\exp[i(\omega t - kx)] + c.c.\} \quad . \tag{3.14}$$

and a magnetic medium polarization P (in A/m; *magnetic* dipole transition assumed) described by

$$P(x,t) = \frac{1}{2}\{i\mathcal{P}(x,t)\exp[i(\omega t - kx)] + c.c.\} \tag{3.15}$$

The following equations for the field envelope $\mathcal{E}$ (x, t) and the polarization envelope $\mathcal{P}$ (x,t) (both are complex quantities) can be derived [3.32, 33]:

$$\frac{\partial\mathcal{E}}{\partial x} + \frac{1}{c}\frac{\partial\mathcal{E}}{\partial t} = -\frac{\gamma}{2}\mathcal{E} + \frac{k}{2\varepsilon_0 c}\mathcal{P} \quad , \tag{3.16a}$$

$$\frac{\partial\mathcal{P}}{\partial t} = -\left[\frac{1}{T_2} - i(\omega_c - \omega)\right]\mathcal{P} + \frac{\varepsilon_0 c}{kT_2}\sigma_c\Delta N\mathcal{E} \quad , \tag{3.16b}$$

$$\frac{\partial\Delta N}{\partial t} = -\frac{1}{2\hbar c}(\mathcal{E}\mathcal{P}^* + \mathcal{E}^*\mathcal{P}) \tag{3.16c}$$

with

- c = ω/k velocity of light in vacuum
- ω = circular pulse carrier frequency
- k = wave number
- γ = linear intensity loss coefficient in m^{-1}
- ε_0 = 8.85×10^{-12} As/Vm electric permittivity of vacuum
- T_2 = transverse relaxation time
- ω_c = circular frequency at line center
- σ_c = $A\lambda^2/4\pi^2\Delta\nu$ induced emission cross-section at line center

A = Einstein coefficient

$\Delta\nu$ = medium line width

λ = radiation wavelength at line center

ΔN = inversion density (in cm^{-3})

$\hbar = h/2\pi = 1.05 \times 10^{-34}$ VAs^2

In (3.16) it has been assumed that the two levels considered are *not* degenerate. The set of equations (3.16) is a special case of the famous "Bloch equations", known from magnetic resonance theory. Two regimes of pulse propagation are distinguished, depending on pulse length τ_p viz. the "coherent" regime, characterized by $\tau_p \leqq T_2$, and the "incoherent" regime, if $\tau_p > T_2$. From (3.16), which are valid in both regimes, the incoherent regime is derived as an approximation for slow polarization changes.

In the incoherent approximation $\partial\mathscr{P}/\partial t$ is neglected compared to $\mathscr{P}/T_2$ and the polarization follows the field quasistatically. Equation (3.16b) then reads

$$\mathscr{P} = \frac{\varepsilon_0 c}{k} \sigma \Delta N \mathscr{E} [1 + i(\omega - \omega_c)T_2] \quad ; \quad \sigma = \frac{\sigma_c}{1 + [(\omega - \omega_c)T_2]^2} \quad . \tag{3.17}$$

Using the expression in (3.16a, c) and introducing the intensity with the well-known relation

$$I = \frac{1}{2} \varepsilon_0 c \mathscr{E}\mathscr{E}^* \tag{3.18}$$

one obtains the following set of equations:

$$\frac{\partial I}{\partial x} + \frac{1}{c}\frac{\partial I}{\partial t} = - \gamma I + \sigma \Delta N I \ , \tag{3.19a}$$

$$\frac{\partial \Delta N}{\partial t} = -2\sigma(I/\hbar\omega)\Delta N \ . \tag{3.19b}$$

These equations are known as the rate equations. They are much easier to solve than the full coherent equations since the number of variables and the number of equations is reduced by one.

It should be noted that only saturation effects on the pulse shape are contained in the rate equations, whereas spectral effects are eliminated. In the small-signal limit therefore, a pulse is not distorted in the rate equation approximation.

It is obvious that the rate equation approximation tends to be the better the longer the pulse length τ_p compared with T_2. However, the validity of the approximation also depends on the amount of saturation by the pulse. This may be appreciated by realizing that at high intensities the Rabi frequency $\mu E/\hbar$ ($\mu = [\varepsilon_o hc\sigma_c/2T_2\omega_c]^{1/2}$ is the magnetic dipole transition moment) may become large compared with $1/T_2$, thus introducing fast polarization changes even at constant intensities. RILEY et al. [3.34] have shown that the fractional error in polarization and consequently in incremental gain for the rate equation approximation is given by

$$\delta_{RE} = \frac{T_2}{\tau_p}(1 + e_p/e_{sat}) \tag{3.20}$$

where e_{sat} is the saturation energy density (for a definition see Sect. 3.3.2), and e_p the instantaneous energy density of the pulse.

In the case of the iodine laser, under most conditions T_2 ranges from 10 to 150 ps and pulse widths τ_p are a few 100 ps or longer. The conditions for the incoherent approximation are therefore approximately satisfied for energy densities up to a few saturation energy densities. It is, nevertheless, advisable to use the coherent treatment for pulse shape calculations. For energy extraction calculations, however, the rate equation approach is entirely satisfactory in most cases.

3.3.2 *Pulse Energy Propagation*

This section treats the incoherent approximation in more detail and shows how the hyperfine spectrum of the iodine laser transition can be taken into account. The rate equations (3.19) can be integrated [3.35] to yield the equation for propagation of the local pulse energy density,

$$e(x) = \int_{-\infty}^{\infty} I(x,t)dt \quad . \tag{3.21}$$

This equation reads

$$\frac{de}{dx} = \sigma\Delta N\, e_{sat}[1 - \exp(-e/e_{sat})] - \gamma e \tag{3.22}$$

with

$$e_{sat} = \frac{\hbar\omega}{2\sigma} \quad .$$

If, as is usually the case in a gas laser, the linear absorption γ can be neglected, this equation can be integrated over the length of the amplifier to yield the often used incoherent saturation formula

$$e_{out} = e_{sat} \ln\{1 + [\exp(e_{in}/e_{sat}) - 1]\exp(\sigma\Delta N\ell)\} \quad (3.23)$$

where e_{in} is the input energy density and ℓ is the amplifier length.

To take the multilevel structure of the iodine atom into account one has to go back to the rate equations and include additional equations for the rates of change of the population densities for the various levels. A closed form solution is then impossible. Fortunately, the magnitude of the relaxation rates between hyperfine levels in many cases allows their contributions to be lumped into the saturation energy density and the system to be treated as a simple two-level system again. This approach has been worked out by FUSS and HOHLA [3.36]. Their treatment involves the definition of a total cross-section σ_{tot}, a homogeneity factor a and a degeneracy factor b: σ_{tot} is the cross-section for stimulated emission relative to the total population in both upper levels (see Sect. 2.1); a is the fraction of the total linewidth which can be considered homogeneous and is therefore available for energy extraction; b takes care of degeneracies and is given by $b = 1 + g_u/g_l$, where g_u and g_l are the effective degeneracies of the upper and lower laser levels. Pulse energy extraction is then described by (3.23), with the saturation energy density being given by

$$e_{sat} = \frac{h\nu}{\sigma_{tot}} \frac{a}{b} \quad . \quad (3.24)$$

In general, experimental situation in terms of pulse width and buffer gas pressure can be approximated by an appropriate choice of the parameters a and b. A few examples are given below.

In the case of a selected mode-locked pulse with a duration of about 1 ns the pulse width is much shorter than the relaxation time between the upper hyperfine sublevels but longer than that between the lower levels. For a pulse with a carrier frequency coincident with the centre frequency of the 3-4 transition and in the case of no overlapping of the lines originating from the F = 3 and F = 2 upper sublevels, one has a = 7/12, b = 1 + 7/24 and a/b = 0.45. Only 45% of the total inversion energy can then be extracted.

If a 3-4 line pulse with a length of about 100 ns, which is long compared with the hyperfine relaxation times in both levels, is fed into an amplifier, one has a = 1 and b = 1 + 12/24 resulting in an energy extraction of 66%. This value is also the upper limit for energy extraction with a multi-line pulse containing frequency components of lines originating from the F = 3 and F = 2 levels.

In an oscillator the value for a/b is between 0.66 and 1 because iodine in the ground state is gradually removed by recombination to the iodide molecule, thus partially eliminating the ground-state bottleneck effect. In the event of no ground-state bottleneck, one has a/b = 1. The result of a pulse energy calculation using (3.23) and a/b = 0.45 is shown in Fig. 3.5.

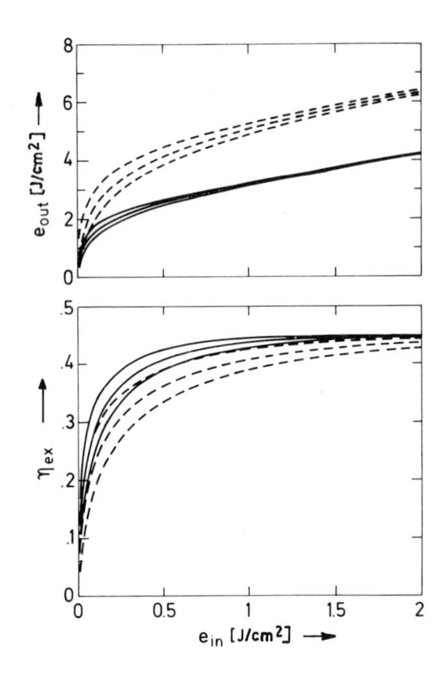

Fig. 3.5. Output energy density e_{out} and extraction efficiency η_{ex} as a function of input energy density e_{in}. (——) e_{st} = 5 J/cm^2; (- - -) e_{st} = 10 J/cm^2. In all cases the three different lines correspond to (going from lower to higher values) A_{ss} = 50, 100, and 300

The effect of the line originating from F = 2 on energy extraction with a 3-4 line pulse has been discussed by BAKER and KING [3.37]. They have shown that the total stored energy of an iodine laser amplifier can be split into two fractions k_1 and k_2, which are extracted at different rates. Two saturation energy densities e_1 and e_2 correspond to the two fractions of energy; e_1 and e_2 are given by the equations

$$e_1 = \frac{4\pi^2\hbar\omega\Delta\nu}{\beta A\lambda^2(1 + g_1/24)}, \quad e_2 = \frac{4\pi^2\hbar\omega\Delta\nu}{\alpha A\lambda^2(1 + g_2/24)} \tag{3.25}$$

where A is the total transition rate probability (= 8 s^{-1}) and where α and β are dimensionless parameters which describe the amount of overlap of the pressure-broadened transitions. They are monotonically increasing with pressure. The quantities g_1 and g_2 are effective degeneracies which depend in a complicated way on α and β. At pressures of up to a few atmospheres of argon the energy formula (3.23) can be used for energy extraction calculations, with an effective saturation energy density being given by

$$e_{sat} = e_1\left(1 + \frac{k_2}{k_1}\frac{e_1}{e_2}\right) . \tag{3.26}$$

This equation is approximately valid in practical regions of interest provided that the output energy density does not exceed e_2 and the pulse carrier frequency ν equals ν_{3-4}.

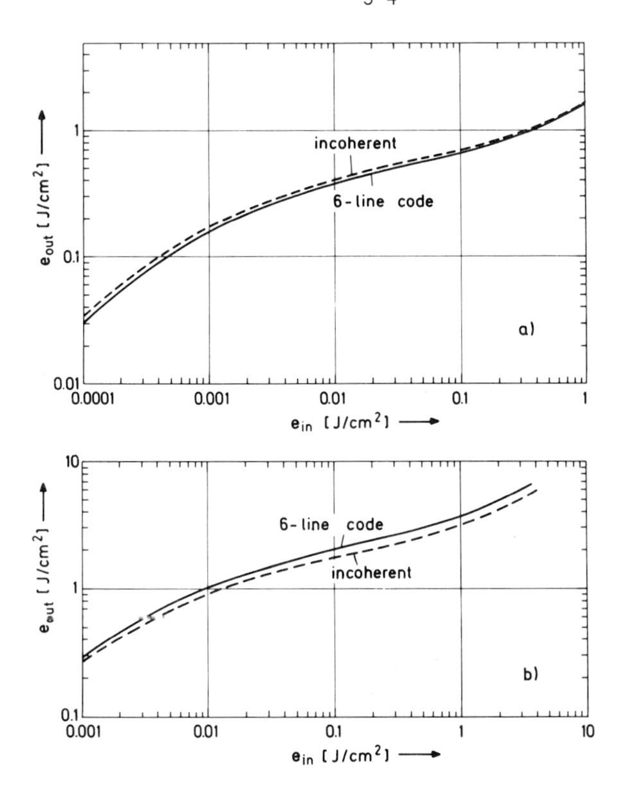

Fig. 3.6. Output vs input energy density of an iodine laser amplifier. Comparison of theoretical prediction from incoherent energy saturation formula ($e_{sat} = 0.45\ h\nu/\sigma_{tot}$) and coherent 6-line code. Input pulse is Gaussian with a width at half maximum intensity of 1 ns. Gain coefficient for both cases $g\ell = 6$ at $\nu = \nu_{34}$ a) $\Delta\nu_p$ = 2 GHz, b) $\Delta\nu_p$ = 10 GHz

At moderate pressures, however, this relatively complicated expression for e_{sat} does not have to be used since the energy saturation formula (3.23) with $e_{sat} = 0.45\ h\nu/\sigma_{tot}$ also gives adequate results. This may be illustrated with the aid of Fig. 3.6. In this figure the output energy density is plotted versus the input energy density for two conditions of pressure broadening. The curve obtained from the simple saturation formula (3.23) is compared with the result of a numerical code which takes into account coherent effects, hyperfine relaxation and energy extraction from all 6 lines [3.34]. It can be seen that at low buffer gas pressure ($\Delta\nu_p$ = 2 GHz) the incoherent treatment overestimates the output energy because the finite linewidth is not taken into account. At high buffer gas pressure ($\Delta\nu_p$ = 10 GHz), however, the incoherent energy saturation formula underestimates the output energy since the contributions of the lines originating from F = 2 are not included. In the example chosen, the error is always smaller than 20%. At higher buffer gas pressures higher errors are expected.

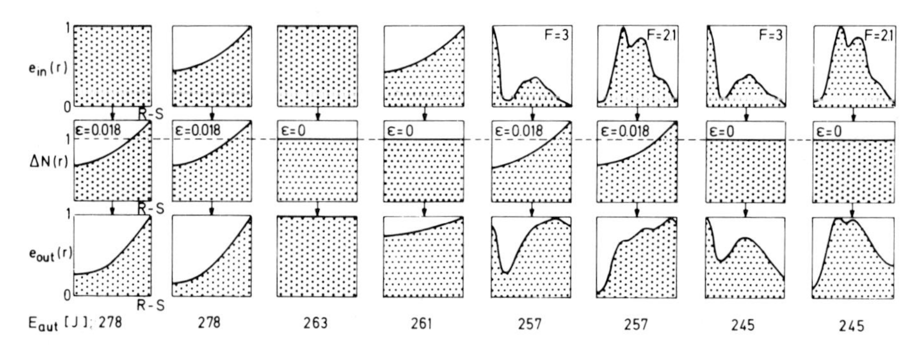

Fig. 3.7. Effect of transverse variation of input energy density and inversion on output energy density and total energy. (F) Fresnel number. (ε) transverse inhomogeneity parameter. (R-S) effective tube radius [see (3.10)]. In all cases E_{in} = 20 J and E_{St} = 1000 J

The incoherent energy saturation formula has been used to study the effect of a transverse variation of both the pulse energy density and inversion density [3.38]. The results are summarized in the diagrams of Fig. 3.7. The upper row gives various examples of profiles for the input energy density (homogeneous, parabolic, Fresnel rings). The inversion profiles shown by the middle row are homogeneous or parabolic. Energy densities and inversions are normalized to the same integrated values. The bottom row shows the resulting output energy density profile for various combinations of input energy density and inversion density profiles. It can also be seen that the output energy is only slightly dependent on the various transverse profiles.

3.3.3 Coherent Pulse Propagation

As mentioned in the introduction, for pulse shape calculations in the subnanosecond region the rate equation approximation is no longer appropriate and the coherent equations have to be used. Because of the complications arising from hyperfine splitting and the various degeneracies of the levels, a fully coherent treatment of pulse propagation in the iodine laser is a formidable task. It involves solution of the Maxwell-Bloch equation for 6 lines, each of which has several degenerate components. The problem is best solved by using the density matrix formalism. The number of levels involved is 36 and therefore the density matrix becomes a 36 x 36 matrix.

Because of these complications various simplifications have been introduced in the published papers on pulse propagation in iodine lasers [3.34,39-41]. Most authors neglect the degeneracies of the various hyperfine levels and treat the hyperfine lines as non-degenerate lines. The error introduced by this summing over magnetic sub-levels is somewhat unclear. Overshoot phenomena are predicted by the "non-degenerate" theory which are washed out when the degeneracy is taken into account. There is also an effect on the predicted energy extraction, as has been discussed by RILEY et al. [3.34]. In the degenerate case there should be some sort of "hole burning" effect within the magnetic sub-level manifold, the transitions with larger matrix elements being saturated first. A non-degenerate theory would therefore predict a slower onset of saturation than would be experimentally observed.

A further simplification can be applied if the frequency of the pulse is coincident with the 3-4 line. This approximation neglects the spectral contributions of all the other lines and retains only the population changes through relaxation from the levels. At moderate buffer gas pressures and intermediate pulse lengths the error of this approximation is smaller than 10%.

If the pulses are not shorter than about 1 ns, the "reservoir effect" of the lower levels can be lumped into an effective degeneracy and the problem treated with a one-line code.

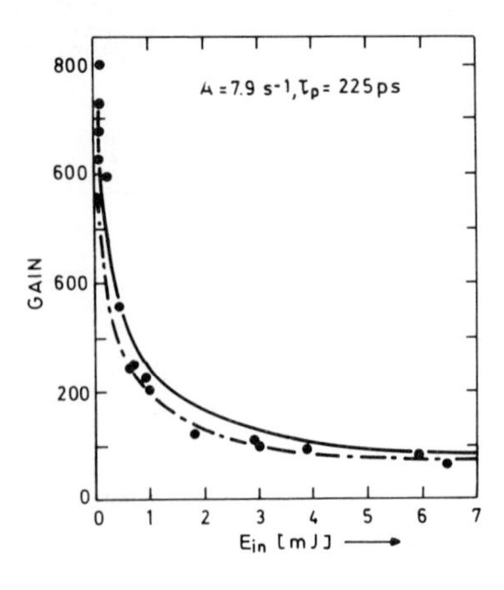

Fig. 3.8. Energy gain vs input energy calculated with coherent 6-line code (nondegenerate theory). (——) pressure broadening coefficient 3.8 GHz/bar. (---) Pressure broadening coefficient 2.3 GHz/bar, adjusted to fit the experimental points [3.34]

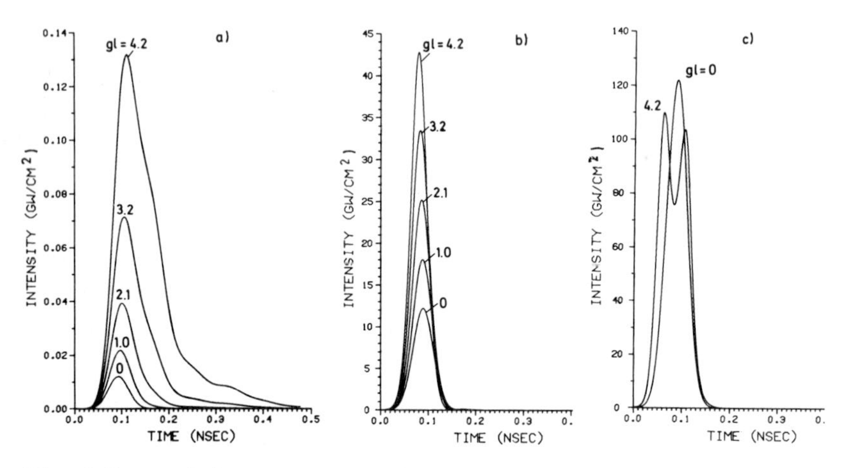

Fig. 3.9 a-c. Pulse propagation in an iodine amplifier calculated with a one-dimensional 6-line code. Gaussian input pulse with τ_p = 50 ps FWHM, e_{st} = 2 J/cm^2, $\Delta\nu$ = 4.5 GHz, a) small signal case, e_{in} = 6.5×10^{-4} J/cm^2, b) saturation, e_{in} = 0.65 J/cm^2, c) very strong saturation, e_{in} = 6.5 J/cm^2

Such a code was used by SKRIBANOWITZ and KOPAINSKY [3.39] to investigate pulse shortening and pulse deformation in iodine laser amplifiers. They found that pulse shortening below a length of about 1 ns is hard to achieve by saturated amplification. Their results agreed well with experimental findings.

An extended one-line code which took into account the reservoir effect of the lower level manifold was used by OLSEN [3.40]. He calculated pulse distortion in a laser amplifier chain. The effect of a saturable absorber incorporated in the chain on the pulse shape and precursor intensity was demonstrated. The predictions of these calculations were later confirmed by experimental results in the ASTERIX III laser amplifier system.

Calculations which take into account all six lines of the hyperfine spectrum have been made by RILEY et al. [3.34]. One of their results, a comparison of theoretical predictions of energy gain with experimental data, is shown in Fig. 3.7. The slight deviations are attributed to the approximation made by neglecting the degeneracies of the hyperfine lines. Results calculated with a slightly adjusted saturation energy density are incorporated in the figure.

Table 3.2. Basic equations for pulse propagation used in coherent 6-line code of UCHIYAMA and WITTE [3.42]

Electric field:	$E(x,t)=\frac{1}{2}\left[\mathcal{E}(x,t)e^{i\Phi}+c.c.\right];\ \Phi=\omega t-kx$
Polarization (Magn.):	$P_{i-j}(x,t)=\frac{1}{2}\left[-i\mathcal{P}^{*}_{i-j}(x,t)e^{-i\Phi}+c.c.\right]$
Sub-level population densities	N_i upper level; $i=2,3$ N_j lower level; $j=1,2,3,4$
Electric field envelope	$\frac{\partial\mathcal{E}}{\partial x}=\frac{k}{2\varepsilon_0 c}\sum_{i,j}\mathcal{P}_{i-j}$; i,j: sum over 6 transitions
Polarization envelope	$\frac{\partial\mathcal{P}_{i-j}}{\partial\tau}=-\left[\frac{1}{T_2}-i(\omega_{ij}-\omega)\right]\mathcal{P}_{i-j}+\frac{\varepsilon_0 c}{kT_2}\sigma_{ij}\,\mathcal{E}\left(\frac{N_i}{g_i}-\frac{N_j}{g_j}\right)\mathcal{P}_{i-j}$
Upper level $i=2,3$	$\frac{\partial N_i}{\partial\tau}=\frac{-1}{T_u}\left[N_i-\frac{g_i}{12}\sum_i N_i\right]-\frac{1}{4\hbar c}\sum_{j=i-1}^{i+1}(\mathcal{E}\mathcal{P}^{*}_{i-j}+\mathcal{E}^{*}\mathcal{P}_{i-j})$
Lower level $j=1\rightarrow i=2;\ j=2\rightarrow i=2.3$; $j=3\rightarrow i=2.3;\ j=4\rightarrow i=3$	$\frac{\partial N_j}{\partial\tau}=\frac{-1}{T_L}\left[N_j-\frac{g_j}{24}\sum_j N_j\right]+\frac{1}{4\hbar c}\sum_i(\mathcal{E}\mathcal{P}^{*}_{i-j}+\mathcal{E}^{*}\mathcal{P}_{i-j})$
Induced emission cross section at line center of the ij-transition	$\sigma_{ij}=\frac{\lambda_{ij}^{2}A_{ij}}{4\pi^{2}\Delta\nu}$
Retarded time	$\tau=t-x/c$

Pulse distortion in an iodine laser amplifier was investigated by UCHIYAMA and WITTE [3.42] also using a coherent 6-line code. The basic equations used in the code are compiled in Table 3.2. The code is one dimensional but allows the carrier frequency of the pulse to be changed or "chirped" through the hyperfine spectrum. Multi-line pulses can also be treated.

In the example shown in Fig. 3.9 the pulse was assumed to have a frequency corresponding to the 3-4 line. As can be seen, in the small-signal regime the pulse is broadened upon amplification because of the finite bandwidth of the gain line. In the saturated region pulse broadening by bandwidth effects and pulse steepening by saturation counteract each other, and the exact parameters determine which dominates. At very high intensities the pulse begins to break up due to coherent effects.

3.3.4 *Application to Amplifier Chains*

The code of UCHIYAMA and WITTE [3.42] was used to investigate various aspects of energy extraction and pulse shaping in a high-power laser amplifier chain. The effects of telescopes, saturable absorbers etc. can be included in the code.

Concerning the energy extraction the calculations revealed that a pulse with a carrier frequency coincident with the 3-4 line will extract 55% of the stored inversion energy from an amplifier when the line of the 3-4 transition is fully saturated. In this case not only the energy stored in the F = 3 sublevel will be extracted but also a part of the F = 2 sublevel energy will be removed because of the overlapping of the two triplets. In an amplifier nearly full saturation will be achieved when the input density is twice as high as the saturation energy density. However, under the realistic conditions of an amplifier chain, where the input energy density is only of the order of the saturation energy density, the extraction efficiency is typically about 50%.

In Fig. 3.10 the propagation of a pulse with a centre frequency at the 3-4 transition is shown at various positions in the ASTERIX III amplifier chain. It is seen that the leading edge of the pulse is considerably steepend in the saturable absorber. In the following amplifier a further reduction of the pulse width takes place because of the smaller amplification of the pulse tail upon saturation.

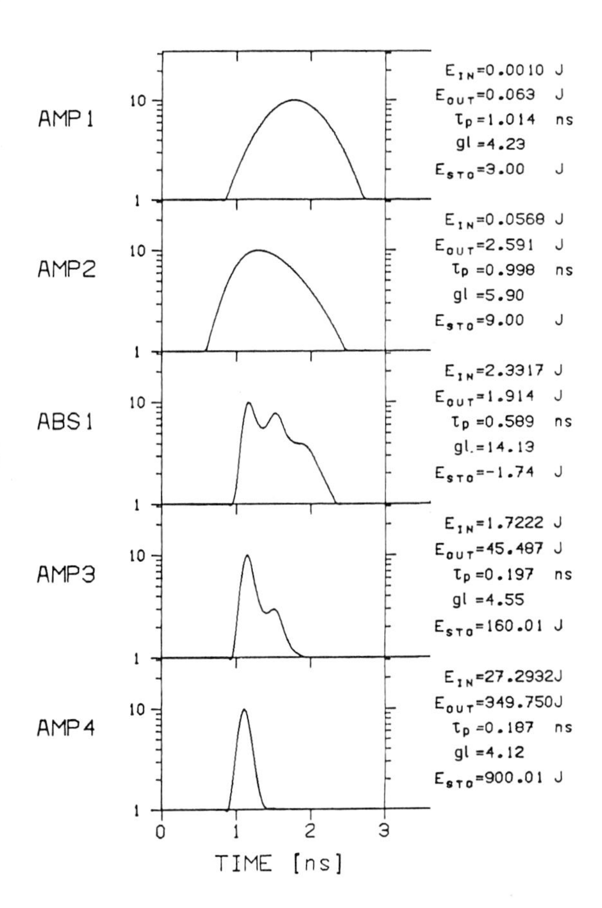

Fig. 3.10. Pulse distortion and energy propagation of a 3-4 line pulse in the ASTERIX III laser system. The chain consists of 4 amplifiers and one saturable absorber. The pulse is slightly attenuated between two units. τ_p = pulse length (full width at half maximum intensity), $\exp(g\ell)$ = small signal amplification at $\nu = \nu_{34}$

The same code [3.42] has been used to predict the pulse energy and pulse width when the carrier frequency of the pulse was varied. The result (Fig. 3.11) shows that the energy is reduced and the pulse elongated when the carrier frequency is detuned from the centre frequency of the 3-4 line.

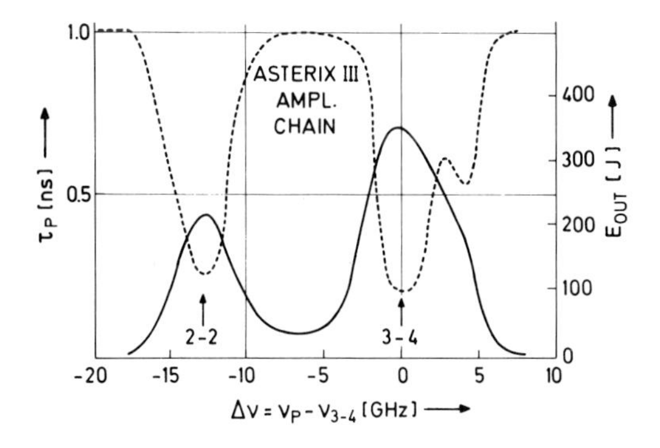

Fig. 3.11. Effect of detuning the carrier frequency of the input pulse to the Asterix III system. (---) pulse length; (——) pulse energy E_{out}

UCHIYAMA and WITTE have also investigated the propagation and energy extraction of a pulse with two carrier frequencies, one coinciding with the centre frequency of the 3-4 transition and the other with the centre frequency of the 2-2 transition. As already mentioned in Sect. 3.3.2, such a pulse could have a higher extraction efficiency than a single-frequency pulse, the theoretical maximum being 66%. The results of the numerical investigations show that it is indeed possible to extract considerably more energy with a multi-line pulse than with a 3-4 line pulse. At a total input energy density of about 0.5 J/cm^2 the extraction efficiency then rises to a value of 60%. Unfortunately, the 2-2 pulse component must precede the other component by several hundred ps for a pulse with a half width time of 1 ns. Otherwise the amplification at the 2-2 line is much smaller than that at the 3-4 line and the 2-2 pulse component becomes unimportant, so that there is little advantage for two-line operation.

The code of UCHIYAMA and WITTE has been used to study the effect of different saturable absorbers in a large laser system such as ASTERIX III (see Fig. 6.1).The main reason for using a saturable absorber in the chain is to reduce the intensity of any precursor pulses or intensities caused by amplified spontaneous emission. However, the absorber also reduces the pulse width (see Fig. 3.12). In the numerical calculations a chain with either

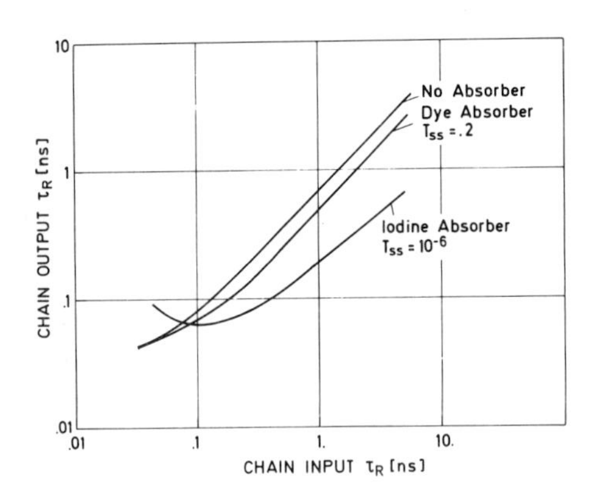

Fig. 3.12. Rise time τ_R of chain output pulse versus rise time of input pulse for different situations concerning the saturable absorber used for prepulse suppression and amplifier decoupling

one narrow-band absorber (T_2~500 ps) placed between the second and third amplifiers or two broad-band absorbers (T_2~50 ps) placed between the second and third as well as between the third and fourth amplifiers was investigated. The strongest pulse compression occurs in the chain with the narrow-band absorber. In both cases, however, the input pulse is considerably longer than the output pulse length.

4. Beam Quality and Losses

There are a variety of mechanisms which change the refractive index of the medium in which the pulse propagates. These changes in the refractive index may lead to a distortion of the wave-front of the pulse, thereby increasing the energy losses of the beam and deteriorating its focusibility. Three different types of mechanisms can be distinguished according to their source and their characteristic time scale.

The first type is induced by the pulse itself and causes refractive index changes due to self-focusing (n_2) or due to saturation of a gain or an absorption line. Self-focusing due to n_2 occurs instantaneously. Saturation is a time integrated change of the refractive index accompanying the transfer of excited iodine atoms ($^2P_{1/2}$) into the ground state ($^2P_{3/2}$) by stimulated emission. The time scale is the pulse length.

The second type results from absorption of the pumping radiation by some constituents of the laser medium adsorbed at the wall of the tube and is responsible for the generation of a shock wave running from the wall of the laser tube towards its axis (a surface effect). In addition, owing to inhomogeneous heating of the laser medium by photolysis of the RI molecules and subsequent exothermic chemical reactions between photolysis fragments, changes of the refractive index of the laser medium will also develop (a volume effect). In both cases the characteristic time scale is given by the ratio d/v (d being the laser tube diamter, and v either the shock wave velocity or the velocity of sound) and ranges from a few microseconds up to several tens of microseconds, depending on the diameter of the amplifier and the medium composition.

The third type is due to the release of heat by the pump source. This heat is partially transferred to the laser quartz tube mainly by radiation and then by conduction and buoyant convection to the laser medium, leading there to turbulence and a vertical gradient of the refractive index which deflects the beam downwards. The damping time of these perturbations is rather long, seconds to minutes, the actual value depending on the size of the amplifier tube, the energy delivered to the flashlamps and the amount of flashlamp cooling.

Finally, two different types of possible losses due to medium turbulence and Mie scattering will be considered and measures to avoid them discussed.

4.1 Pulse-Induced Gradients of the Refractive Index

4.1.1 Self-Focusing Due to n_2

Wave-front distortions of this type only become important for short pulses ($\leqq$ 0.5 ns) and are due to an intensity-dependent refractive index obeying the relation

$$n_r = n_0 + n_2\langle E^2\rangle = n_0 + \hat{\gamma}I \qquad (4.1)$$

where n_0 is the normal refractive index for a low-intensity beam, $\langle E^2\rangle$ denotes the time average of the electric field E over a cycle and is proportional to the light intensity I, and n_2 and $\hat{\gamma}$ are related by the expression

$$\hat{\gamma} = \frac{n_2}{\varepsilon_0 c n_0} \qquad (4.2)$$

where $\varepsilon_0 = 8.86 \times 10^{-12}$ As/Vm is the permittivity of free space and $c = 3 \times 10^8$ m/s the vacuum speed of light. Values of $\hat{\gamma}$ for the media of interest for the iodine laser are given in Table 4.1. Dispersion effects in the wavelength range from 0.6 to 1.3 μm have been neglected. The $\hat{\gamma}$ values of CF_3I and C_3F_7I have been estimated using the bond additivity model [4.4]. Although these values are rather large they have little effect on the self-focusing properties of the laser medium which are dominated by the buffer gas since the concentration of the perfluoroalkyl iodides is small. Self-focusing due to n_2 becomes effective when the pulse has a transverse intensity variation. In this case the high-intensity zones of the pulse move more slowly than the low-intensity zones, thereby distorting the wave-front. If the intensity profile has its maximum on the axis and smoothly falls off towards the edge, the beam will be focused as a whole. If the intensity profile is, however, not smooth, but exhibits intensity ripples caused by diffraction from the beam-limiting apertures or small dust particles on the optical surfaces, these

Table 4.1. $\hat{\gamma}$ values of some gases in the wavelength range from 0.6 to 1.3 μm (dispersion neglected); BK7 added for reference

Gas	$\hat{\gamma} \times 10^{19}$ [cm^2/W]	Comment	Ref.
air (1 bar, 300 K)	7 ± 3	from $\chi^{(3)}(-3\omega,\omega,\omega,\omega)$	4.1,2
He (")	0.5	theoretical value	4.3
Ar (")	4 ± 1	from K_m	4.3
CO_2 (")	7 ± 3	from $\chi^{(3)}(-3\omega,\omega,\omega,\omega)$	4.1
SF_6 (")	8 ± 2	from K_m	4.3
CF_3I(10mbar, 300K)	0.4 ± 0.2	from $\chi_n^{(3)}(-2\omega,0,\omega,\omega)$	4.4[a]
C_3F_7I(")	0.8 ± 0.4	"	
BK7	3600 ± 400		4.6

[a] $\chi^{(3)}$(C-I bond) estimated from extrapolation of the known $\chi^{(3)}$ values for the C-F, C-Cl and C-Br bonds; $\chi^{(3)}$(C-C bond) estimated using the molar Kerr constant of CH_4 and C_2H_6 [4.5]

Conversion Formulas Used in Table 4.1

$n_{2,esu} = 12\,\pi\chi^{(3)}_{1111}\ (-\omega,\omega,\omega,-\omega)\ N/n_0$ for isotropic molecules [4.7,9];

$\chi^{(3)}_{1111}$ in esu/molecule or atom; N number denstiy per cm^3.

$$\text{Assumptions (see also [4.8]): } \chi^{(3)}_{1111}\ (-\omega,\omega,\omega,-\omega) \cong \begin{cases} \chi^{(3)}\ (-2\omega,0,\omega,\omega) \\ \chi^{(3)}\ (-3\omega,\omega,\omega,\omega) \\ 81\ K_m\ /\ 24\ \pi\ N_A \end{cases} .$$

The $\chi^{(3)}$'s are third-order non-linear optical susceptibilities. For their meaning see references quoted. K_m is the molar Kerr constant in esu-units, N_A Avogadros number.

$n_{2,SI} = n_{2,esu} \times 10^{-8}/9\ [m^2/V^2]$; $\hat{\gamma}$ according to (4.2) with $n_2 = n_{2,SI}$.

---

intensity fluctuations will be enhanced when the pulse propagates through the system. This process may ultimately break up the beam into a large number of small filaments [4.10]. In any case, the focusibility of the beam is adversily affected by the self-focusing phenomena, making it impossible to get a diffraction-limited focal spot. Moreover, since the focusing behaviour is time dependent - the leading and trailing edges of the pulse have other axial focus positions than the centre portion (beam zooming) - it is difficult to eliminate this aberration by a phase correction device.

A quantitative measure of the beam quality in this respect, taken at a position z in the amplifier chain, is given by the so-called beam breakup integral B defined by [4.10]

$$B(z) = \frac{2\pi}{\lambda} \int_0^z \hat{\gamma}(z')I(z')dz' \qquad (4.3)$$

where λ is the pulse wavelength, and I the peak intensity of the pulse, usually the value on the laser axis z. As can be seen from (4.3) the self-focusing effect due to n_2 is cumulative, i.e. it adds up when the pulse runs through the amplifier chain. Theory and experiment have shown that there exists a critical value of B which should not be exceeded [4.10-13]. Otherwise small-scale instabilities with their catastrophic consequences will develop, setting in for "noisy" beams at $B \geqq 2.5$ and for "clean" beams at $B \geqq 4$. The growth of these small-scale instabilities can be avoided by means of spatial filters [4.11] which remove the high spatial frequency components (most damaging ripples) from the angular spectrum of the beam, thereby resetting B = 0 for these components. Thus, whenever B approaches its upper limit in an amplifier chain, a spatial filter is necessary. This technique is widely employed in Nd lasers, such as SHIVA and OMEGA where many spatial filters in a single amplifier chain are the rule [4.10]. It should, however, be noted that in contrast to the small-scale instabilities the whole beam self-focusing cannot be reduced by spatial filters. For this effect B is not reset to zero after each spatial filter, so that it adds up throughout the amplifier chain. For SHIVA [4.12], for example, total values for B of 12 are typical (at 100-ps pulse duration) which corresponds to a wave-front distortion of two wavelengths. As a consequence, the focal spot diameter cannot be better than 5 to 6 times the diffraction-limited value [4.13]. The whole beam self-focusing thus presently represents one of the factors limiting the achievable power from any glass-laser system operating in the 50-100 ps regime.

For the iodine laser the situation is basically more favourable than for solid-state lasers because it is a gas laser and does not require as much glass thickness in the optical beam line.Only passive components such as windows, polarizers, Faraday rotators and Pockels cells are required for the iodine laser. Because of the longer beam path (ASTERIX III: 150 m [4.14]; see also Chap.6) it has, however, to be confirmed whether the gaseous media, some of which are at high pressure, make a noticeable contribution to the B integral. For the present performance of the ASTERIX III system (300 J/0.3 ns), B is approximately equal to 2 at the exit of the last amplifier [4.14] so that no spatial filter is needed in the chain. The contribution of the gaseous media to the total value of B amounts to ~30%, this being almost exclusively due to the long distance of 80 m in air between the third and fourth amplifiers.

Since ASTERIX III under present conditions is operated at a relatively low intensity level, it is clear that if an iodine laser system were to be operated at higher intensity levels, more attention must be paid to the self-focusing problem. This conclusion holds for the glass components as well as for the gaseous media. In the latter case both the propagation in the free space and in the active medium has to be considered. For example, in an improved version of the ASTERIX III system [4.14] with a projected output power of 2.5 TW (500 J/0.2 ns; comparable to ARGUS with 2.3 TW/beam [4.11]) the following contributions to the B integral are expected: glass 3.3; free space 0.7 to 1.4 (0.7 with, 1.4 without a beam expander between the third and fourth amplifiers); amplifying medium 0.4 with argon as buffer gas and 0.8 with SF_6 as the buffer gas. As a consequence, two spatial filters, the first between the third and fourth amplifiers and the second behind the fourth amplifier will be needed to keep the small--scale instabilities from growing. The total B will be between 4.4 and 5.8, so that the focal spot diameter can be estimated to be 2 to 3 times its diffraction-limited value [4.13], the deviation being caused by the whole beam self-focusing. Since the increase of B per amplifier is clearly below 2.5, the diameter of the main amplifiers is controlled by the damage threshold of the AR coating of the exit window. The layout of the ASTERIX III system is thus fluence limited. This statement holds for pulse durations down to 50 ps.

To summarize, for short-pulse operation (≤500 ps) an iodine laser working primarily in the saturation regime has to use properly staged spatial filters in order to control small-scale self-focusing resulting both from the glass and the gaseous media (air, buffer gas). The system design remains fluence limited down to pulse durations of ~50 ps. The number of spatial filters needed will be less than half of the value of a Nd laser of comparable performance. For pulses ≧0.5 ns, self-focusing due to n_2 becomes unimportant in an iodine laser, so that in this case no spatial filters are needed in order to control self-focusing but may be desirable for other purposes (such as amplifier decoupling and image relaying) to maintain a smooth beam profile [4.10] (see also Chap.7).

4.1.2 Saturation Phenomena

A necessary condition for any efficient high-power laser is operation in the saturation regime. The shape of the wave-front is affected when either the intensity of the pulse or the inversion has a transverse variation. The response of the medium is not instantaneous, but is instead time integrated in the sense that the changes in the refractive index become larger as more iodine atoms are transferred from the excited state ($^2P_{1/2}$) to the ground state ($^2P_{3/2}$). Owing to the time integrated nature of the process, the trailing edge of the pulse is more affected than its leading edge, thus causing time-dependent behaviour of the focus pattern.

Saturation of a gain or absorption line not only changes the pertinent anomalous index of refraction, but also the non-resonant part of the total refractive index resulting from all the other transitions. This is due to the fact that the polarizability of the excited iodine atoms is slightly larger than that of the ground-state iodine atoms. The accompanying change of the refractive index is always negative for a gain line and always positive for an absorption line, in contrast to the change of the refractive index due to anomalous dispersion, which can alter the sign within a gain or absorption line, depending on the carrier frequency of the pulse and the linewidth of the laser medium (superposition effects due to the hyperfine structure of the iodine atom). Under favourable conditions both effects may cancel each other.

The anomalous dispersion (subscript "r" for resonant) is treated first. Of interest is the phase difference $\Delta\phi_r$ between an on-axis ray and a ray at the beam edge. It is thereby assumed that the edge ray undergoes small-signal amplification whereas the on-axis ray saturates the laser medium. The maximum possible value of $\Delta\phi_r$ occurs when the on-axis portion of the beam fully saturates the medium over the entire amplification length. In this case $\Delta\phi_r$ is equal to the phase shift of the edge ray due to anomalous dispersion which can be written as (in rad like B)

$$\Delta\phi_r = -\frac{\lambda^2 A_{tot}}{4\pi^2\Delta\nu}\left(N_u - \frac{1}{2}N_\ell\right)\ell\left\{\frac{7}{24}\sum_{j=2}^{4}\frac{A_{3j}}{A_{tot}}\frac{x_{3j}}{1+x_{3j}^2} + \frac{5}{24}\sum_{j=1}^{3}\frac{A_{2j}}{A_{tot}}\frac{x_{2j}}{1+x_{2j}^2}\right\}$$

with

$$x_{ij} = \frac{\nu - \nu_{ij}}{\Delta\nu/2} \qquad (4.4)$$

where N_u and N_ℓ are the population densities of the upper ($^2P_{1/2}$) and lower ($^2P_{3/2}$) laser levels. The meaning of the other symbols is as in Chap.2. Equation (4.4) has been evaluated using the results of [4.15].

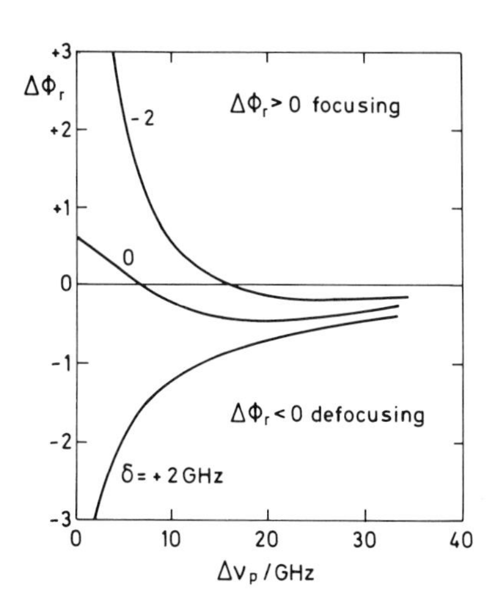

Fig. 4.1. Resonant wave-front distortion $\Delta\phi_r$ versus medium linewidth $\Delta\nu_p$ • $\delta = \nu - \nu_{34}$ detuning of the pulse carrier frequency ν from the centre frequency ν_{34} of the 3-4 transition. $\ell(N_u - 1/2\ N_\ell) = 4 \times 10^{19}/cm^2 \hat{=} 6\ J/cm^2$

In Figure 4.1 $\Delta\phi_r$ is plotted versus the medium linewidth $\Delta\nu_p$ with the detuning of the pulse carrier frequency ν from the centre frequency ν_{34} of the 3-4 transition as a parameter. Only for zero detuning is the wave-front distortion due to saturation negligible. Because of this fact the pulse carrier frequency should always coincide with the centre frequency of the 3-4 line.

The predictions of $\Delta\phi_r$ made with (4.4) are in qualitative agreement with the results of [4.16] where a 2-D computer code in the paraxial approximation was used to explore possible self-focusing effects due to anomalous dispersion (the non-resonant contribution was not considered there). As reported in [4.16] strong pulses are focused for $\Delta\nu_p \leqq 12$ GHz whereas the opposite holds for $\Delta\nu_p \geqq 12$ GHz, i.e. defocussing occurs. Moreover, the changes of the shape of the wave-front are of the order of $\lambda/10$ or less, as calculated above ($\lambda/10$ corresponds to $\Delta\phi_r \sim 0.6$).

The phase difference $\Delta\phi_{nr}$ accounting for the wave-front distortion due to the non-resonant part of the refractive index is treated under the same assumption as $\Delta\phi_r$, i.e. full saturation of the laser medium by the on-axis ray. One then obtains

$$\Delta\phi_{nr} = -\frac{(2\pi)^2 \ell}{\lambda} (\hat{\alpha}_{I^*} - \hat{\alpha}_I) \frac{2}{3} (N_u - \frac{1}{2} N\ell) \tag{4.5}$$

where $\hat{\alpha}_{I^*}$ and $\hat{\alpha}_I$ are the polarizabilities of the iodine atom in the excited and ground states ($\hat{\alpha}_I = (9 \pm 2) \times 10^{-24}$ cm^3, [4.17]). The difference $\Delta\hat{\alpha} = \hat{\alpha}_{I^*} - \hat{\alpha}_I$ has been measured in [4.18] where a value of $(3 \pm 1) \times 10^{-26}$ cm^3 was found. With $\ell(N_u - 1/2\ N_\ell)$ corresponding to 6 J/cm^2 as in Fig. 4.1, $\Delta\phi_{nr}$ becomes -0.3 ± 0.1 (defocusing) and thus negligibly small. This finding is supported by the results of [4.16] where the measurements of the wave-front distortion were satisfactorily explained by the calculations considering only the anomalous dispersion.

4.2 Refractive Index Gradients Due to Absorption of Pump Light

The phenomena to be discussed in this section (in Sect. 6.2.3 referred to as intensity-independent wave-front distortions) result from the absorption of the pump light occurring at the surface (shock wave) and in the volume (acoustic waves). Perturbations of the first kind propagate with the shock wave velocity a_s, and those of the second kind with the speed of sound v_s. The characteristic time within which the shock wave disturbs the homogeneity of the laser medium is hence the laser tube diameter d divided by a_s. The characteristic time of the acoustic waves is given by ℓ_s/v_s where ℓ_s denotes the length scale of the perturbed volume. In the following it is assumed that ℓ_s equals the tube diameter d, i.e. the acoustic pertubations extend over the entire volume of the laser cell. This is the usual situation in case of inhomogeneous pumping. In order to keep the influence of both types of pertubations as small as possible, the pumping time T_p must be small compared with the ratios d/a_s and d/v_s.

In this context it should be briefly mentioned here that changes of the refractive index also instantaneously arise from the dissociation of RI molecules since the added polarizabilities of the radical and the free iodine atom are not equal to that of the parent molecule. This difference was experimentally determined in [4.18] for C_3F_7I. A refractive index change of ~5 x 10^{-8} was observed for a density of 10^{17} dissociated C_3F_7I molecules per cm^3. Unless the inversion profile is very inhomogeneous (e.g. edge inversion more than twice as big than the on-axis inversion), the wave-front distortion resulting from this gradient of the refractive index is negligible. In the amplifier mode the same holds for the wave-front perturbations due to the refractive index changes arising from the recombination process R + I → RI and the quenching process I* + M → I + M [4.18], if the pumping time is short.

The gasdynamically induced phase aberrations of the pulse are much easier to correct than those caused by the pulse itself because the former are static and do not change over the pulse length. Things are especially favourable when the refractive index either rises or falls monotonically from the edge towards the centre of the laser tube. In this case it is only the curvature of the wave-front that is altered, but the brightness can be maintained. This situation is typical of the case of the inhomogeneous heating of the laser medium by photodissociation. The case of the shock wave is more difficult to deal with because here the gradients of the refractive index are rather strong, as will be discussed in the next section.

4.2.1 Shock Wave

There are numerous papers [4.19-25] in which it has been shown that a shock wave originates at the wall of the laser tube and runs towards its centre. Measurements of the shock wave velocity a_s [4.19-22,25] have yielded values of 1.2 to 2 times the speed of sound v_s determined from the medium conditions prior to photolysis. The larger values were found in media without any buffer gas where the medium temperature may have become quite large. If in this case the local speed of sound is taken as the reference speed, the ratio a_s/v_s is then reduced to values between 1.2 and 1.4. These are also found in media strongly diluted with buffer gas where a temperature rise is negligible.

A weak dependence of a_s on the pump flux in (W/cm^2) has been observed in [4.23]. Trebling the pump energy increased a_s by 10%. Since in the other experiments referenced above, the pump flux varied over several orders of magnitude, but in all of them similar values for a_s were found, it therefore has to be concluded that a_s is only weakly dependent on the pump flux[1].

The most important mechanism responsible for the generation of the shock wave (pyrolysis, although a possible mechanism [4.23], is not important here since it can be suppressed by a sufficient amount of buffer gas what is always the case in high-power amplifiers) is the adsorption of molecular iodine onto the laser tube walls and its abrupt liberation by the flashlamp light (~500 nm) [4.19]. In addition to the molecular iodine there may also be other pumplight absorbing layers at the inner wall tube (see Chap.5, contamination problems): metal iodide powder, carbon deposits resulting from RI photolysis at wavelengths <200 nm [4.25] or hydrocarbon layers arising from reactions of oil vapor (sources: vacuum pump, vacuum grease, inadequate cleaning procedure of the laser tube prior to assembly) with photolysis products. All of these layers can produce a shock wave when they are irradiated with pump light.

However, there are measures that can be taken to avoid the formation of these layers (for details see Chap.5) so that they will not be further considered here. The only question which remains to be answered is whether the build-up of an I_2 layer can be prevented. This is possible when the laser tube is evacuated between shots to a pressure of $\sim 10^{-6}$ mbar as has been demonstrated in [4.25]. For a big laser system, however, this is not a technically feasible solution. In order to achieve a reasonable repetition rate and to limit the medium consumption, a gas circulation-regeneration system has to be used (see Chap.5). In this case the deposition of I_2 on the inner laser tube wall is unavoidable.

In order to decide the question whether an interaction of the beam with the shock wave can be tolerated, the refractive index gradient across this disturbance must be known. For the buffer gases of interest (argon, SF_6), it turned out to be 4×10^{-5} cm^{-1} [4.19].

In mixtures with a *high helium content* and using pump pulses with a *gently* rising leading edge (~100 μs with a total length of 300 μs), dn/dr at the end of the pump pulse may be considerably lower than the value of 4×10^{-5} cm^{-1} [4.19,26], which is typical of the first appearance of the shock wave and for buffer gases of high molecular weight. Owing to reflec-

---

[1] For the strength of the shock wave this statement does not strictly hold. If the shock wave velocity increases by 10%, the density jump across it is raised by 20% (valid for $1 \leq a_s/v_s \leq 1.5$).

tion losses (for t_p = 300 μs, d = 1 cm, 20 reflections of the shock wave at the laser tube wall are possible in helium at $a_s = 1.3 \times 10^5$ cm/s), the refractive index gradient may be reduced still further. The authors of [4.26] claimed that under these conditions interaction of the pulse with the shock wave is tolerable, leading to a beam which is twice diffraction limited.

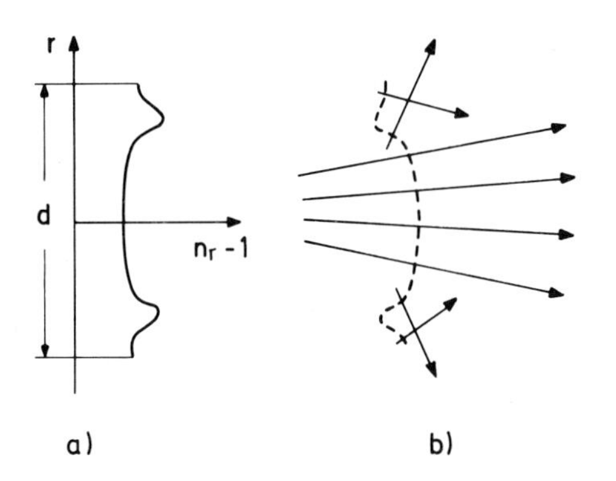

Fig. 4.2a,b. Interaction beam-shock wave (schematically). (a) Refractive index profile, (b) wave-front (---) and beam directions (——) after passage through the amplifier

Since for high-energy storage amplifiers helium is not an attractive buffer gas because of its low broadening coefficient and long pulse durations are undesirable for various reasons (see next sections), the large value for dn/dr of 4×10^{-5} cm^{-1} has to be accepted. This means, for example, that in an amplifier only 1 m long, the divergence of the portion of the beam which has been hit by the front of the shock wave increases by 4 mrad (see Fig. 4.2). The angular frequency spectrum of the beam is thus considerably broadened by the interaction of the beam with the shock wave. Since the high-frequency components generated are very inconvenient for target experiments, they either have to be taken out of the beam by spatial filtering or to be avoided altogether by choosing a beam diameter such that no interaction of the beam and shock wave is possible. In any case, the existence of the shock wave means an energy loss since only a portion of the energy stored in the laser tube is available for the pulse to be amplified. The requirement to tolerate only a small fractional loss ΔE/E (E energy stored in the entire tube volume) can be used to establish a relationship for the maximum pump duration T_p :

$$T_p \leq \frac{d}{4a_s} \left\{ \frac{\Delta E}{E} - \varphi \frac{\ell}{d} \right\} \tag{4.6}$$

where d is the tube diameter, ℓ the tube length and φ the beam divergence (unperturbed). For $\Delta E/E = 0.1$, $\varphi = 10^{-4}$ rad, $\ell = 10$ m, d = 20 cm and argon as the buffer gas ($a_s = 450$ m/s) the upper limit for the pump duration is 12 µs.

4.2.2 Inhomogeneous Heating

The refractive index changes associated with inhomogeneous heating of the laser medium are typical of that part of an amplifier tube which has not yet been reached by the shock wave. These index changes are usually rather smooth. Their occurrence is conditional on a spatially varying photolysis rate (number of RI dissociations per unit volume and unit time). This is the normal situation because it is very difficult to illuminate a volume homogeneously under the conditions pertinent for high-energy storage. This statement holds for flashlamp-pumped systems as well as for amplifiers pumped by open high-current discharges ("exploding wires"). In the first case the flashlamps are usually located outside the tube confining the laser media so that the inversion drops from the edge towards the centre of the tube (see, for example, [4.27]). In the second case the situation is reversed when the discharge takes place in the middle of the laser medium. The inversion is then highest close to the centre of the tube and falls off towards the edge [4.28]. Configurations where many open discharges are placed close to the periphery of the laser tube are also in use [4.29]. The inversion profile is then similar to the flashlamp case. The heating of the laser medium results from the fact that in each dissociation process about 30% of the excitation energy of 4.8 eV is converted to heat. This results from the conservation of energy. The energy needed to crack the C-I bond is 2.3 eV and about 1 eV is transferred to the excited iodine atom. The remaining energy of 1.5 eV is firstly converted to vibrational-translational energy of the radical and translational energy of the iodine atom. The translational energy of the radical and the iodine atom is quickly distributed among all molecules or atoms of the laser medium via collisions. The thermalization of the vibrational energy may be somewhat delayed if a molecular buffer gas such as SF_6 or CO_2 is used since these molecules become vibrationally excited by collisions with hot photolysis fragments. The time scale of this delay is a few microseconds at buffer gas pressures around 1 bar [4.18]. When the gasdynamic time scale d/v_s is much larger, the delayed heating effects have little influence on the development of the perturbation of the refractive index. This is assumed to be the case in the following considerations.

Besides heating of the gas by some fraction of the dissociation energy, there is an additional heating due to chemical reactions such as $2\,R \rightarrow R_2$ where the C-C bonding energy of 4.2 eV is set free, and due to the quenching of I* yielding an energy of 1 eV/atom. These contributions also have to be taken into account. (Only the amplifier mode of operation is considered here.)

When the pump energy is inhomogeneously deposited in the laser medium, the heat production due to all the processes mentioned above is also inhomogeneous. Thus a temperature gradient as well as a pressure gradient are established which sets the gas, originally at rest, into motion, thereby changing the gas density and the index of refraction. These disturbances propagate with the speed of sound v_s and become stronger with time. To keep their influences as small as possible the pumping time T_p should be small compared with d/v_s.

Determination of the refractive index changes following the onset of the pump light is rather complicated when the medium is optically thick with respect to the pump radiation and/or strong temperature rises occur. In such cases only a numerical calculation can give the correct answer [4.30]. Fortunately, under the conditions usually prevailing in an amplifier chain, an analytical approach is also possible [4.18,20,31] where the following restrictions are made: medium optically not thick, fraction of the dissociated RI molecules ≦25% (no bleaching) and relative temperature rises $\Delta T/T_0 \leqq 0.1$ (T_0 being the temperature prior to photolysis) due to strong dilution of the RI molecules with buffer gas and/or moderate pumping.

In this case it turned out that for the determination of the refractive index changes it is not necessary to follow the behaviour of each species of the medium separately. Instead, it suffices to consider only the average gas density ρ of the medium, which is related to the wavefront distortion $\Delta\phi_{ih}$ by [4.20]

$$\Delta\phi_{ih} = \frac{2\pi\ell}{\lambda}(n_{r,o} - 1)\left\{\left(\frac{\rho}{\rho_o}\right)_{centre} - \left(\frac{\rho}{\rho_o}\right)_{edge}\right\} \tag{4.7}$$

where the subscript "o" refers to the state of the medium prior to photolysis and $n_{r,o}$ is the unperturbed index of refraction given by

$$n_{r,o} = 1 + \frac{1.5}{N_A}\sum_i r_i N_i \ . \tag{4.8}$$

Here $N_A = 6.023 \times 10^{23}$ particles/mol is Avogadro's number, r_i and N_i are the molar refraction in cm^3/mol and the number density per cm^3 of the species i.

The calculation of the gas density perturbation is greatly simplified if isochoric heating is assumed [4.18,31]. This is a good approximation as long as $t < d/2v_{s,o}$ holds. If this condition is met, the density perturbation is given by [4.18,31]

$$\frac{\rho - \rho_0}{\rho_0} = \frac{(\gamma - 1)}{\gamma} \frac{v_{s,o}^2}{p_0} \int_0^t \left(\frac{1}{r} \frac{\partial q}{\partial r} + \frac{\partial^2 q}{\partial r^2}\right) dt'^3 \tag{4.9}$$

where γ is the ratio of the specific heats of the medium at constant pressure and constant volume, p_0 the medium pressure and q the heat function. Equation (4.9) is only valid in the volume which has not yet been reached by the shock wave. If this disturbance is not present, the boundary condition of zero velocity at the tube wall requires the existence of a rarefaction wave moving inwards with the speed of sound v_s. In this case (4.9) is again only correct in the region not yet influenced by the rarefaction wave. The refractive index changes occurring across this wave are also so strong that this region cannot be used in high-power amplifiers.

The heat function q is related to the photolysis rate w(r,t) (RI dissociations per cubic centimeter and second) according to

$$q(r,t) = w(r,t)\{\varepsilon_p + \varepsilon_{cc}[1 - \exp(-t/t_D)]\} \tag{4.10}$$

where $\varepsilon_p = 1.5$ eV and $\varepsilon_{cc} = 4.2$ eV are the heat releases of the dissociation and dimerization ($2R \rightarrow R_2$) processes[2]. The heat contribution of the latter reaction is only approximately accounted for since it strictly depends on w in a non-linear manner. However, after a delay time of the order of t_D the dimerization closely follows the time and spatial behaviour of w. The time delay t_D is different for the various alkyl iodides and approximately given by

$$t_D = 1/2\sqrt{k_D \hat{w}} \tag{4.11}$$

---

[2] The quenching contribution has been neglected in (4.10) since it is assumed that the pumping time is short enough.

where k_D is the rate constant of the dimerization process (see Table 2.5) and $\hat{w}$ the space-time averaged photolysis rate defined by $2T_M(\pi d^2/4)\hat{w}= 2\pi\int\int w(rt)rdrdt$. Here T_M is the time it takes the pump light to reach its maximum value. At $\hat{w} \cong 10^{22}$ cm^{-3} s^{-1} (which is a typical value for ASTERIX III type flashlamps and RI pressures), t_D is 2 μs for CF_3I, 6 μs for for i-C_3F_7I and 30 μs for t-C_4F_9I.

Since bleaching is neglected w(r,t) simply reads [4.18,20,31]

$$w(r,t) = w_s\, g(t)\, h(r) \tag{4.12}$$

where $w_s = m\hat{w}$ holds. The value of m depends on the choice of g(t) and h(r) which are normalized functions. The function g(t) accounts for the time dependance of the pump light and h(r) for its local variation. The form of h(r) can be experimentally derived from small-signal amplification measurements since h(r) is proportional to the inversion profile. To a good approximation h(r) can be represented by an even power series in r, thus

$$h(r) = \sum_{0}^{j_E} c_{2j}\left(\frac{r}{d/2}\right)^{2j} \quad . \tag{4.13}$$

Introducing (4.9-13) in (4.7), the wave-front distortion $\Delta\phi_{ih}$ is given by

$$\Delta\phi_{ih} = -48\pi\,\frac{\ell}{\lambda}\,\frac{w_s\varepsilon_p}{d^2}\,\frac{(\gamma - 1)r_{tot}}{M_{tot}}\sum_{2}^{j_E} j^2 c_{2j}\left(\frac{r}{d/2}\right)^{2j-2}\int_0^t g(t')$$

$$\cdot\left\{1 + \frac{\varepsilon_{cc}}{\varepsilon_p}\left[1 - \exp\left(-\frac{t'}{t_D}\right)\right]\right\}dt'^3 \tag{4.14}$$

where r_{tot} and M_{tot} are the molar refraction and molecular weight of the laser medium, respectively. From (4.14) several conclusions can be drawn:

a) For an inversion profile purely quadratic in r (c_4, c_6, all zero), no wave-front distortion results, $\Delta\Phi_{ih} = 0$. This occurs when the product $\sigma_{max}N_{RI}d$ equals 2 as was shown in [4.18] (σ_{max} is the peak absorption cross-section, see Table 2.4). For the ASTERIX III type amplifiers, $\sigma_{max}N_{RI}d = 3$ is chosen in order to get a sufficient pump light absorption. In this case, terms up to the sixth order in r have to be retained in (4.13) leading to [4.31]

$$h(r) = 1 + 0.5\left(\frac{r}{d/2}\right)^2 + 0.2\left(\frac{r}{d/2}\right)^4 + 0.1\left(\frac{r}{d/2}\right)^6 \cdot \tag{4.15}$$

The refractive index corresponding to such a pump profile is proportional to the second derivative $(1/r)(d/dr)(rdh/dr)$ of $h(r)$ and contains both a quadratic and quartic term in r. The quadratic term (lens) represents an increase in the beam divergence. It thus shifts the focal spot position and slightly increases the focal spot size. The quartic term mainly acts on the focal spot size which is enlarged.

b) The role of the buffer gas is contained in the quantity $(\gamma-1)r_{tot}$ / M_{tot} which can thus be used to minimize the optical disturbances. Since the alkyl iodides are strongly diluted with buffer gas in high-power amplifiers, r_{tot} and M_{tot} are dominated by the buffer gas properties. A compilation of data for some buffer gases is made in Table 4.2.

Table 4.2. Gasdynamic figure of merit of various buffer gases

Gas	$r[cm^3/mol]$	M[g/mol]	γ	$(\gamma-1)r/M$ $[cm^3/g]$
He	0.56	4	1.67	0.094
Ar	4.5	40	1.67	0.075
CO_2	7.2	44	1.30	0.049
SF_6	13.4	146	1.09	0.0085
C_4F_8	20.5	200	1.06	0.0060

Table 4.2 shows that the commonly used argon is not the best choice; SF_6 and C_4F_8 appear more attractive. There are, however, situations where these compounds cannot be used. These occur in large-diameter amplifiers employing a circulation system and operated at pressures ≧4 bar. Here the cold trap temperature may become so low that SF_6 or C_4F_8 condense. Quenching of I* by these compounds may be another reason to rule them out. This is, however, only to be expected at pressures of several bar and pumping times exceeding 20 μs (see Sect. 2.3.5 and Table 2.5).

The gasdynamic model as outlined above has been experimentally confirmed by several authors [4.18,20,31]. The measured optical disturbances could be satisfactorily reproduced by employing (4.10-15). These equations may thus also confidently be used to predict the wave-front distortion in high energy-storage amplifiers. For example, for the last amplifier of the ASTERIX III system [$d=17$ cm, $\ell=800$ cm, $w_s=3\hat{w}=2\times10^{22}/cm^3s$, $t_D=6$ μs, $T_M=5$ μs, 4 bar argon, $g(t)=(t/T_M)^2\cdot\exp(-t^2/T_M^2)$, $h(r)$ according to (4.15)], $\Delta\phi_{ih}$ at t=12 μs and r=0.4 d is calculated from (4.14) to be -0.8. This has a negligible effect on the beam quality which was experimentally found to be close to the diffraction limit. This supports the theoretical calculations.

Generally, for amplifiers with external flashlamp pumping and an inversion profile according to (4.15), a rule of thumb can be deduced from (4.14) stating that the optical disturbances due to inhomogeneous heating are unimportant as long as the relation between pumping time T_p and the diameter d,

$$T_p \leqq 0.03\ d/v_s \quad , \tag{4.16}$$

is met. This condition leads to similar values for T_p [see (4.6)] resulting from the shock wave or, if absent, from the rarefaction wave, when a_s is replaced by v_s.

Equation (4.14) is also applicable to amplifiers with pump sources embedded in the laser medium, either flashlamps or open high-current discharges [4.29,32-34]. In the latter case the heat function is probably not as simple as described by (4.10). The presence of radiation below 180 nm makes the photolysis process and the chemical kinetics much more complicated [4.35] and increases the heating of the laser medium even further so that possible wave-front distortions have to be carefully monitored.

This section is concluded by briefly mentioning the small-scale intensity fluctuations with transverse dimensions of up to a few millimeter observed in the radiation pattern of an iodine laser oscillator pumped by an open discharge [4.36] or by flashlamps [4.18, 4.37]. These disturbances are not caused by non-uniform deposition of pump energy, but by the laser radiation itself. If the optical field is spatially inhomogeneous, this will lead to an inhomogeneous concentration of the ground--state iodine atoms generated from excited iodine atoms by induced emission. The fast recombination reaction I + R → RI and the dimerization reaction 2R → R_2 which are exothermic with 2.3 eV and 4.2 eV then lead to an inhomogeneous heating of the laser medium and thus to a modulation of the refractive index of the gas. It was shown in [4.38-41] that these gasdynamic perturbations can reach a steady state so that stationary stimulated light scattering becomes possible. Since the build-up time of the stimulated waves takes a few μs, this effect is not harmful to nanosecond pulses.

4.3 Refractive Index Gradients Due to Heat Release of the Pump Source

As already mentioned this type of refractive index change is of concern for repetition rate operations of ≦10 min/shot only and is thus especially important for the layout of the flashlamp and quartz tube cooling system.

4.3.1 Beam Deflection

The heat released by the flashlamps is partially absorbed by the quartz tube and then transferred to the laser medium via conduction and buoyant convection whereby a vertical temperature gradient is caused in the laser medium. Assuming that the pressure is constant everywhere in the laser medium, the refractive index behaves in an opposite manner to the temperature: it decreases in the upward direction so that the beam is deflected downwards. According to (4.8) and the relation $p = NkT$ (k Boltzmann constant, T gas temperature) the gradient of the refractive index can be written as

$$\frac{dn_r}{dy} \simeq -\frac{1.5}{d}\frac{r}{R}\frac{p}{T}\frac{\Delta T}{T} \tag{4.17}$$

where R is the universal gas constant, r the molar refraction of the laser medium and $\Delta T > 0$ the temperature difference between top and bottom of the tube. Using ray optics the beam deflection angle reads

$$\theta = \frac{dn_r}{dy}\,\ell \simeq -\frac{3}{2}\frac{\ell}{d}\frac{r}{R}\frac{p}{T}\frac{\Delta T}{T} \quad . \tag{4.18}$$

For a temperature difference ΔT of only 1 K, a buffer gas pressure of 4 bar argon ($r = 4.5$ cm^3/mol) and a typical value of 40 for the ratio ℓ/d $\theta = 2 \times 10^{-4}$ rad is obtained. For a distance of 20 m between two consecutive amplifiers, a vertical beam displacement of 0.4 cm thus occurs. This example clearly demonstrates the necessity of a well-designed cooling system for the flashlamps and the quartz tube; otherwise the beam will be so strongly deflected that after a few shots an amplifier chain will be completely misaligned.

4.3.2 Turbulence

In addition to the changes of the refractive index n_r described in the previous section, there are other variations of n_r arising from temperature fluctuations within the turbulent gas induced by the regeneration system (see Sect. 5.2.1) and buoyant convection. Since the characteristic dimension Λ of these random inhomogeneities is much smaller than the beam diameter d, the beam acts as though it is passing through a medium with an extinction coefficient, i.e. the beam suffers a loss [4.42]. The scattered part of the pulse emerges as an *incoherent* beam of increased divergence, typically of angular spread λ/Λ as opposed to λ/d for the unscattered part of the beam. Since one typically has $(d/\Lambda) \gg 10$, the scattered radiation is completely lost when the pulse has travelled a few meters. The angular spectrum of the beam thus does not have to be stripped of high-frequency components by means of a spatial filter or, in other words, the wave-front of the beam remains unaffected by the microturbulence of the laser medium.

In this context a short note on the problem of air turbulence seems appropriate. It may play a role when the amplifiers are separated by long distances. Since the length scale of this kind of turbulence is usually of the order of the beam diameter, the beam will be strongly affected: its optical axis is tilted and its angular frequency spectrum is broadened, both in a statistical manner, i.e. varying from shot to shot. Thus, as a consequence air turbulence has to be avoided either by putting the perturbation sources into a different room or by shielding the beam from these disturbances by means of tubes.

4.4 Losses

Two kinds of losses are dealt with in the following. The first refers to medium turbulence and the second to Mie scattering. Both losses are especially important in laser systems designed for high repetition rate operation.

Losses resulting from Rayleigh, Raman or Brillouin scattering are usually negligible [4.43,44]. Only in the final air path from the exit of the amplifier chain to the target chamber there might be sufficient Raman gain to convert an appreciable amount of laser radiation to Raman-shifted radiation if this distance turns out to be rather long ($\geq$25 m). However, by pumping the final air path down to 100 mbar or by filling it with helium or argon, stimulated scattering can be avoided. Strong Raman scattering between two consecutive amplifiers within a chain is very unlikely since the distances over which high intensities occur are too short.

4.4.1 Beam Losses Due to Medium Turbulence

As already outlined in Sect. 4.3.2, microturbulence of the laser gas acts upon the beam as if it were passing through a medium with an extinction coefficient. In our case interest is restricted to temperature fluctuations caused by heat transfer from the quartz tube to the laser medium, mainly by buoyant convection, and by the regeneration system (see Sect. 5.2.1). The disturbances arising from the latter source are only important when it is running and until shortly after it has been switched off. This source will thus only be active in high repetition rate operation. It is assumed that these fluctuations are randomly distributed and are on a scale that is small compared with the beam diameter d. In this case the scattering theory of SUTTON [4.42] may be used to calculate the extinction coefficient

$$\bar{\alpha} = 2k^2 \Lambda \langle \Delta n_r^2 \rangle \tag{4.19}$$

where $k = 2\pi/\lambda$; Λ is the turbulence scale size and $\langle \Delta n_r^2 \rangle$ the mean square fluctuation of the refractive index. With due consideration of (4.8), $\bar{\alpha}$ reads

$$\bar{\alpha} = 2\left(\frac{3\pi r N}{\lambda N_A}\right)^2 \Lambda \left(\frac{\overline{\Delta T}}{T}\right)^2 \tag{4.20}$$

where r is the molar refraction and N the number density of the laser medium. $\overline{\Delta T} = \{\langle \Delta T^2 \rangle\}^{1/2}$ signifies the root-mean-square temperature fluctuation. An estimate of the turbulence macroscale Λ can be made on the assumption that it should be close to the smallest dimension of the regeneration system, i.e. a few millimeters (cold trap; these small dimensions are necessary for efficient I_2 separation). On the other hand, the smallest turbulence length scale (Kolmogorov microscale) turns out to be about 0.1 mm [4.45]. So, $\Lambda \sim 1$ mm appears to be an acceptable choice. The temperature fluctuation $\overline{\Delta T}$ is supposed to be ~0.1 K. With these values for Λ and $\overline{\Delta T}$ we find $\bar{\alpha} \leqq 10^{-4}$/cm at 5 bar SF_6 and $\bar{\alpha} \leqq 10^{-5}$/cm at 5 bar argon. This means that in an amplifier 10 m long the beam will suffer a loss of ≦10% in the case of SF_6 and ≦1% in the case of argon.

In summary, scattering losses due to microturbulence of the laser medium may become important for long amplifiers ($\ell \geqq 10$ m) operated at pressures ≧4 bar, but only in the case of SF_6.

4.4.2 Beam Losses Due to Mie Scattering

It is an experimental fact that in the iodine laser medium flashlamp pump light produces small, solid particles which can easily be seen in the light of a He-Ne laser [4.44]. Up to now the composition and origin of these particles are not clear and several explanations are equally probable. The particles may result from interaction of atomic iodine generated by the photodissociation of I_2 and RI molecules with the inner surface of the quartz tube [4.46] whereby small SiO_2 particles are formed with diameters equal to or smaller than a few micrometres. They may also be condensed molecular iodine or an iodine-oxygen compound, I_2O_5. Despite these uncertainties it has been proven that these aerosols cause Mie scattering of the beam and according to [4.44] a concentration as low as 10^3 particles/cm^3 is sufficient for a 10% loss at an amplifier length of 10 m. Comparable losses were found in the third amplifier of the PLASTERIX laser [4.44] immediately after a shot. With the regeneration system of this laser, 10 min were required before the transmission went back to the loss--free state; at shorter circulation times only incomplete recovery could be achieved. In this particular example it took a considerable time to deposit the aerosols outside the laser tube.

No specific conclusions can be drawn from this example since the recovery behaviour depends on the layout and dimensions of the regeneration system and must be experimentally determined in individual cases. But it has to be kept in mind that Mie scattering may be a serious loss mechanism and should be considered in each amplifier design, especially in the case of high repetition rate operation, when there is little time to remove the aerosols from the active zone.

4.5 Summary: Wave-Front Distortion and Losses

In the preceding sections of this chapter various sources distorting the pulse wave-front have been analyzed in detail. All of them can be controlled in such a way that they will have little effect on the beam quality.

For short pulses ($\leq$500 ps), the dominating phenomenon is self-focusing due to n_2 occurring in passive components such as glass, buffer gas and air. Spatial filters are needed in order to avoid the growth of small-scale instabilities. However, the effect of n_2 on the laser performance is not as strong as in solid-state lasers. This is - among other things - reflected by the fact that the layout of an iodine laser remains fluence limited down to ~50-ps pulse durations. Saturation phenomena occurring at any pulse length can usually be neglected unless the carrier frequency of the pulse is detuned from the 3-4 line. In this case careful analysis of possible wave-front distortions is necessary.

The problem of the shock wave is best solved if any interaction between it and the beam is avoided. This requires short pumping times $\leqq 0.03\ d/a_s$ in order to keep the losses small. Wave-front distortions resulting from the inhomogeneous heating of the laser medium by the absorption of pump light and by exothermic chemical reactions are negligible when the inversion at the centre and at the edge of an amplifier do not differ from each other by more than a factor of 2 and the pumping time is kept below $0.03\ d/v_s$; otherwise this effect must be monitored carefully.

Finally, for repetition rates higher than 15 min/shot a cooling system is necessary to remove the heat released by the flashlamps; otherwise downward beam deflection will be induced, making the alignment of the system impossible. Beam losses due to medium turbulence are only to be expected for long amplifiers ($\geqq 10$ m) when molecular buffer gases are used, for example, SF_6 or CO_2. Beam losses due to Mie scattering have to be checked for in high repetition operation, when there is little time left to remove the aerosols from the laser tube.

5. Design and Layout of an Iodine Laser System

The preceding chapters have been devoted to the physical principles of the iodine laser, the generation and amplification of short pulses, and the scaling laws of a single amplifier stage. This chapter now deals with the technical aspects and possible versions of an iodine laser system such as can be built at present for its main field of application, namely laser fusion research.

Such a laser has to meet the following requirements. Firstly it should be capable of delivering pulse energies of up to a few kilojoules per beam at an energy density loading of up to several joules per square centimetre with pulse lengths ranging from several hundred picoseconds to a few nanoseconds. In addition, the beam should have an almost diffraction-limited quality, a temporally smooth pulse shape, and a directional shot-to-shot stability not allowing focus position fluctuations higher than small fractions of the focal spot size. Typically this corresponds to angular stabilities of the order of microradians. Furthermore, the prepulse energy or average power has to be below a level such that sensitive targets are not destroyed before the main pulse strikes them ($E_{Pr} < 1$ mJ, $P_{Pr} < 100$ W).

In addition, a fusion research laser should afford reliable and reproducible operation with sufficiently high pulse rates (for research requirements preferably about one shot every 30 min). At the same time, economic aspects require that the efficiency of converting pump energy into laser pulse energy should be as high as possible.

The difficulty of satisfying all these requirements is determined by the physical and technical properties of the laser medium and the pump source. In general, these properties do not allow all of the requirements to be satisfied at the same time. The design of a laser system therefore has to be based on a compromise between requirements imposed by laser-fusion experiments and the need to minimize the cost of both construction and subsequent operation.

5.1 Design of an Amplifier Chain

The performance of an iodine laser is based on the storage and subsequent release of inversion energy. The essential components of such a laser include the oscillator and the amplifiers with their optical pumping systems and the equipment for laser medium regeneration. Further components serve for selecting the pulse to be amplified, for beam expansion, for optical isolation of the amplifiers from each other, for prepulse suppression and for the protection of sensitive laser components from damage due to laser light retro-reflected from the target.

To design a laser system at the lowest cost for a specified level of system performance, several steps are required. First of all, models for simulating system components have to be established and tested experimentally. In addition, the cost data of the components have to be scaled with size and specifications. Finally, when the regime of operation is suitably defined and system requirements have been established, a computer model for the design of an optimized system can be developed. Such a model for an iodine laser, however, does not exist at present. This is due to the fact that models simulating system components have not yet been defined for all relevant components, and also that the cost data of specific iodine laser components, such as amplifiers, are lacking.

Models for describing the performance of some of the iodine laser components are, however, available. They deal with the energy extraction from a single amplifier stage and the flashlamp circuit configuration including the reflector geometry. These models have been developed by HAGEN [5.1] and are based on his models for the simulation of Nd-glass laser systems.

In the following discussions, only first-order design criteria for constructing an iodine laser can, therefore, be defined. These criteria will be based on the physics of the pumping, storage and extraction of inversion energy and hence they deal mainly with amplifiers and their scaling in a chain. Since these devices together with their capacitor banks constitute the most elaborate and costly components of the laser, and since they are, in addition, the major active parts, they primarily determine the physical geometry of the entire laser chain.

An amplifier chain consists of pre- and main amplifiers. The preamplifiers amplify the oscillator pulse to such an energy level that the following main amplifiers can be operated close to saturation fluences. The formal distinction between these two types of amplifiers is given by the fact that the output energy density or output fluence (J/cm^2) of preamplifiers is relatively small, whereas in main amplifiers the maximum output fluence e_m permitted by the damage threshold of components will usually be achieved.

Before the design criteria of an amplifier chain can be discussed, however, the scaling and the efficiency relationships of a single amplifier need to be described.

5.1.1 Scaling and Efficiency Relationships of Amplifiers

Large aperture amplifiers are the most costly components of a laser system. They have, therefore, to be operated at the highest system fluences to extract their stored energies efficiently and to minimize the beam diameters (and hence the costs of components). The maximum fluence value e_m permitted by the damage threshold of the most sensitive components, the AR coatings of the amplifier exit window, is 3-4 J/cm^2 for a pulse length of 1 ns. This is half of the damage threshold value e_d specified in Sect. 5.3.3. Since the damage threshold of coatings scales roughly as the square root of the pulse length, for longer or shorter pulses the maximum fluences have to be increased or reduced according to the relation given in [5.2]. If graded index surfaces are used, the maximum incident energy density e_m can be raised to a value of 6 J/cm^2.

Simple first-order scaling laws for the design of a large aperture amplifier have already been established in Sect. 3.2.4. For external flashlamp pumping, these are: The effective amplifier diameter d_{eff} which covers the area not perturbed by shock waves scales according to

$$d_{eff} = 2\sqrt{E_{out}/\pi e_m} \quad [cm] \quad . \tag{5.1}$$

The geometrical amplifier diameter d is related to the effective amplifier diameter d_{eff} by

$$d = d_{eff} + 2a_s T_p + \varphi\ell \tag{5.2}$$

where a_s is the velocity of the shock wave (for Ar: $a_s \leqq 450$ m/s) and T_p the effective pumping time, which is in present installations $T_p \cong 3$ µs for $d \leqq 5$ cm, $T_p \cong 10$ µs for $5 \leqq d \leqq 20$ cm and $T_p \cong 15$ µs for $d > 20$ cm. φ is the beam divergence (full angle, in general, $\varphi \leqq 1$ mrad). The length ℓ of an amplifier is defined by

$$\ell = e_{st}/up_{RI} \quad [cm] \tag{5.3}$$

where e_{st} is the stored inversion energy density, which ranges for the main amplifiers between 6 and 7 J/cm^2, u the specific inversion energy density measured to be u = 1 mJ/mbar cm^3, and p_{RI} is the partial pressure of the alkyl iodide (RI pressure). Its value is determined by the geometrical amplifier diameter d according to

$$p_{RI}d = 200 \quad [\text{mbar cm}]. \tag{5.4}$$

The pressure of the buffer gas then depends on the species of gas employed and on the required small signal amplification factor at the stored inversion energy density (3.7). When argon is used as a buffer gas, its value can be drawn from Fig. 3.3.

In the case of the preamplifiers, the RI pressure and the pressure of the buffer gas are determined by the same relations applicable to the main amplifiers. Since, however, in the preamplifiers the maximum allowable fluence will not be achieved, their effective diameter cannot be defined by a simple scaling law. This diameter is chosen such that it accomodates the oscillator output pulse diameter and the effective diameter of the first main amplifier ($0.5 \leqq d_{eff} \leqq 2.5$ cm). The length of a preamplifier is also defined by (5.3). It depends on the RI pressure and the stored inversion energy density, which for preamplifiers is in the range of 2-6 J/cm^2.

The iodine laser amplifier efficiency is defined by the ratio of the electrical energy stored in the capacitor bank divided by the optical energy extracted by the pulse. This efficiency depends on two processes: the pumping process, which converts electric energy into stored inversion energy; and the extraction process of the stored inversion energy by the pulse to be amplified. The extent to which the efficiencies of both processes can be optimized at minimum cost will be investigated in the following section.

First the pumping process will be considered. The discussion will be restricted to flashlamp pumping because this technology has hitherto proved to be the most suitable one at an efficiency comparable with or higher than those of the other methods described in Sect. 2.2. Flashlamp pumping efficiency is impaired by several loss processes. The conversion of electrical energy stored in the capacitor banks E_{el} into UV radiation overlapping the iodine absorption band around 270 nm depends mainly on the physics of the discharge process in the flashlamps. The potential for improvements of this process is quite limited (see Sect. 2.2.2).

Not all of the light emitted by the flashlamps is coupled into the amplifiers. Its amount depends on the pumping configuration, which is defined by the shape and the reflectivity of the reflectors, and the positioning of both the reflectors and the flashlamps. The measures for optimizing these quantities are described in Sect. 5.2. Not all of the pumping light overlapping the 270 nm absorption band and radiated into the amplifiers will be absorbed by the laser medium. The amount absorbed is determined by the relation of the RI pressure to the amplifier diameter. The absorption process cannot be maximized, otherwise excessive RI pressures would be required, thus resulting in excessively inhomogeneous inversion profiles in the amplifiers (Sects. 3.2.3 and 4.2).

The relation between the electrical energy E_{el} to be stored in the capacitor bank and the total inversion energy $(E_{st})_{tot}$ stored in the full amplifier volume after completion of the pumping process is given by

$$(E_{st})_{tot} = \eta_{el} E_{el} \quad . \tag{5.5}$$

where η_{el} describes the efficiency for the conversion of the total stored electrical energy into inversion energy. Its value depends on the amplifier diameter. For $d \leqq 20$ cm, it increases slowly with increasing diameter. Its value is described by the empirical relation

$$\eta_{el} \approx 7.5 \times 10^{-3}(1 - 0.7/d) \ . \tag{5.6}$$

For $d \geqq 20$ cm, η_{el} is practically constant. It has a value of $\eta_{el} = 7.5\ 10^{-3}$.

Not all of the stored inversion energy is available for the pulse to be amplified. Shock wave interactions and beam expansion reduce the full amplifier area $F_{tot} = \pi d^2/4$ to the effective area $F_{eff} = \pi(d-2a_sT_p-\varphi\ell)^2/4$. The ratio

$$K = F_{eff}/F_{tot} \quad , \tag{5.7}$$

ranges between $0.5 \leqq K \leqq 0.8$ for amplifiers with diameters $2.5 \leqq d \leqq 30$ cm (for Ar $a_s \leqq 450$ m s^{-1}, $\varphi \leqq 1$ mrad; $T_p \cong 3$ µs for $d < 5$ cm, $T_p \cong 10$ µs for $5 \leqq d \leqq 20$ cm and $T_p \cong 15$ µs for $d > 20$ cm). Also the requirement for minimizing the shock wave losses restricts the use of full pumping energy. The pulse has to pass through the amplifier before the pumping process has been completed. The fraction of the stored inversion energy available for the pulse in the total amplifier area is then described by

$$P = (E_{st})_{T_p}/(E_{st})_{tot} \tag{5.8}$$

where T_p is the effective pumping time. For amplifier diameters $d \leqq 20$ cm, P has a value of 0.75, and for larger diameters, a value of 0.8.

Since the inversion energy E_{st} available for the pulse to be amplified is $E_{st} = K\,P\,(E_{st})_{tot}$ and $E_{st} = e_{st}\,F_{eff}$ where e_{st} is the stored energy density, the total electrical pumping energy is described by

$$E_{el} = e_{st}F_{eff}/KP\eta_{el} \ . \tag{5.9}$$

The design of a single amplifier can now be carried out, provided that the values of the maximum output energy density e_m, of the effective pumping time T_p, of the required output energy $E_{out} = e_{out}F_{eff}$ and of the stored inversion energy denstiy e_{st} are given. This energy density has the following form:

$$e_{st} = (e_{out} - e_{in})/\eta_{ex} \ . \tag{5.10}$$

The parameters on e_{out}, e_{in} and η_{ex} can be specified when the entire amplifier chain has been designed and the relation between the input energy density e_{in} and the extraction efficiency η_{ex} is known.

The dependence of the extraction efficiency on the input energy density has already been calculated in Sect. 3.3.2 for an input pulse having a frequency coincident with the centre frequency of the 3-4 transition, which is the frequency of the pulse usually emitted by an oscillator. The results are displayed in Fig. 3.5. The incoherent saturation formula (3.23) has been used in this case. The energy stored in the F=2 upper sublevel has not been included and the maximum extraction efficiency is therefore only 45%. Under the conditions of an actual amplifier chain, however, overlapping of the lines originating from the F=2 and F=3 upper sublevels takes place, and the energy stored in the F=2 sublevel will be partially extracted. Extraction efficiencies of up to 60% can then result.

To calculate the actual extraction efficiencies as a function of the input energy density, the six-level code described in Sect. 3.3.3 has been used. These calculations have been performed for a 1-ns pulse whose carrier frequency coincides with the centre frequency of the 3-4 transition at a small-signal amplification of 100, which is a reasonable upper bound for an amplifier incorporated in a chain. The parameters are the stored inversion energy densities of 4.7, 7.0 and 9.3 J/cm^2 respectively. The calculated curves are plotted in Fig. 5.1. As shown, they differ only slightly from one another. At an input energy density of 0.5 J/cm^2, the extraction

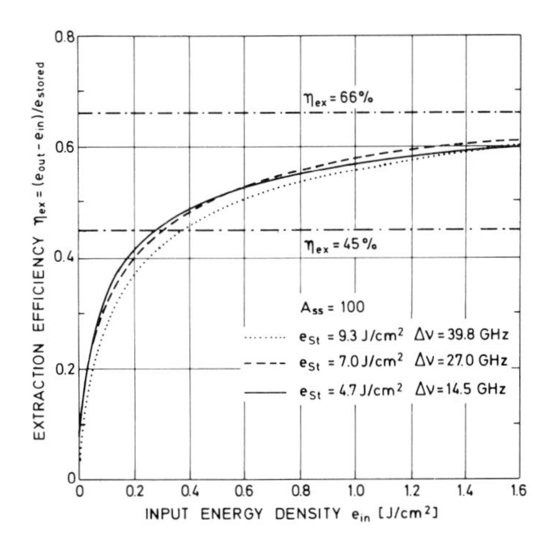

Fig. 5.1. Extraction efficiency vs input energy density (single pass) at stored inversion energy densities of 9.3, 7.0 and 4.7 J/cm^2 (A_{SS} = 100)

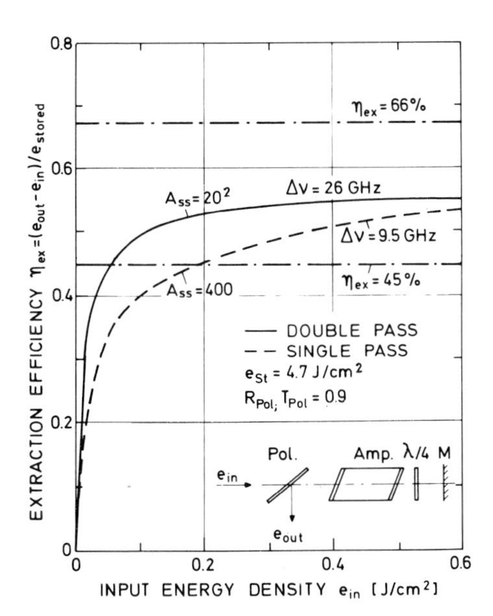

Fig. 5.2. Extraction efficiency vs input energy density for single (A_{SS} = 400) and double pass (A_{SS} = 20^2) at a stored inversion energy density of 4.7 J/cm^2 [reflectivity and transmission of the polarization-sensitive mirror (Pol): R = T = 0.9]

efficiency reaches a value in the range of 50%, while an input energy density of 1.5 J/cm^2 will raise it to the 60% level.

According to the relation $e_{st} = (e_{out} - e_{in})/\eta_{ex}$ the maximum output energy density of e_m = 3.5 J/cm^2 permitted by the damage threshold of AR coatings will be achieved with an input energy density of 0.5 J/cm^2 at a stored inversion energy density of 6.0 J/cm^2, and with an input energy density of 1.5 J/cm^2 at a stored inversion energy density of 3.3 J/cm^2. These two cases do not violate the restriction set by the pressure limitation for the buffer gas.

As already described in Sect. 3.2.2, the buffer gas pressure should not significantly exceed values of 6 bar in large aperture amplifiers ($d \geqq 8$ cm) because of the problems associated with the handling of high pressures in large volumes. This requirement restricts the maximum storable energy density to about 6.5 J/cm^2 at a small signal amplification of 100 with argon used as a buffer gas.

When an amplifier is operated in a double-pass geometry, high extraction efficiencies can be obtained at lower input energy densities. With an input energy density as low as 0.1 J/cm^2, an extraction efficiency of about 50% can be achieved. The double pass geometry is shown in the insert of Fig. 5.2. The entrance and exit beams are separated by a dielectric polarizer after double pass through a $\lambda/4$ plate.

In order to avoid parasitics, the single pass gain ($\ln A_{ss}$) should be only half that used in the single-pass scheme. Compared to this geometry the stored inversion energy density in the double pass case therefore has to be decreased correspondingly, assuming the buffer gas pressure is the same for both geometries. For a double pass small-signal amplification of 400, the stored inversion energy density has to be reduced to a value of 4.7 J/cm^2 at a maximum buffer gas pressure of 6.8 bar. For these conditions, the dependence of the extraction efficiency on the input energy density was calculated by the six-level code (Sect. 3.3.3). The results are shown in Fig. 5.2. The strong reduction of the input energy density by the double-pass method in order to achieve the same η_{ex} is clearly demonstrated. At an input energy density of only 0.3 J/cm^2, an extraction efficiency of 55% is obtained, and thus the maximum output energy density will be 2.9 J/cm^2. If the small-signal amplification and hence the stored inversion energy density have to be reduced, the maximum output energy density will correspondingly decrease.

The factor limiting the storage of a sufficiently high inversion density in a double-pass amplifier is the gain reduction requirement. In principle, it can be relaxed if a saturable absorber of the Jul 2 type (Sect. 5.3.4) is placed between the amplifier and the quarter-wave plate. However, the numerical analysis of such a configuration reveals that, owing to the insufficient large-signal transmission of the absorber, the performance of the double-pass scheme can only then be significantly improved, when the pulse passes through the amplifier mainly in the small-signal regime and through the saturable absorber in the saturated regime. In this case the pulse energy amplification factor nearly reaches the relatively high value of the single pass, small-signal amplification A_{ss}. The saturable absorber losses are more than compensated for by the enhancement of the total small-signal amplification of the amplifier allowed by the saturable absorber. The double-pass technique combined with a saturable absorber is therefore ideally suited for amplifiers working in the small-signal regime. For an application in the transition regime or the large-signal regime, the saturable absorber must be removed. The use of the double-pass scheme can only then be recommended when high extraction efficiencies are required at low input energy densities, and the output energy density need not attain the highest level as in the case of the large-aperture amplifiers.

Before applying the double-pass method it should, however, be checked whether the benefit achieved justifies the increased effort. This is because the advantage of higher extraction efficiency at a low input energy density will be partially offset by an increased outlay for equipment and a decrease in the ease of beam handling.

5.1.2 Criteria for the Design of an Amplifier Chain

On the basis of the efficiency studies described in the previous section, first-order design criteria for an amplifier chain will now be defined. The efficiency of the amplifier chain depends primarily on the pumping and extraction efficiencies of its various amplifiers. Their pumping efficiencies will, however, not affect the scaling of the chain. They influence only the costs of the pumping arrangements including the capacitor banks. To minimize the cost of these components, the pumping efficiency should be optimized to such an extent that the cost for construction and maintenance should be lowest, while affording high system reliability.

Preamplifiers. As the energy extraction efficiency depends on the amplifier input energy density and on the stored inversion energy density at a given small-signal amplification, this efficiency defines the scaling of an amplifier chain consisting of preamplifiers and main amplifiers. The oscillator pulse energy (in the 1-mJ range) should be raised in the preamplifiers to such an energy level that the following main amplifiers can be operated at high energy extraction efficiencies. The design criteria for the main amplifiers are based upon the conservation of this high extraction efficiency along the chain.

The operation of the preamplifiers is characterized by the fact that full medium saturation is in general not achieved, and that the maximum output energy density e_m will not be obtained. In an optimum preamplifier, the small-signal gain should be maximized at a modest level of the stored inversion energy density. The limitations on the maximum sustainable small-signal amplification are mainly imposed by optical feedback between adjacent amplifiers. For amplifiers with the feedback provided by spatial separation, the maximum tolerable small-signal amplification A_{ss} is approximately 100 per amplifier. For amplifiers with better isolation, as afforded by a Pockels cell or a saturable absorber, 2 - 3 times higher values can be tolerated.

The energy amplification in a preamplifier is described in a sufficiently good approximation (see Fig. 3.6a) by the incoherent saturation formula (3.23). Two preamplifiers in general provide sufficient amplification to reach saturation in the first main amplifier. Theoretically preamplifiers should preferably be operated in the double-pass geometry. In practice, however, only the second amplifier can be driven in this mode. This is due to the fact that for pulses in the nanosecond region, the first pass cannot deliver the power density required to saturate the dye absorber incorporated in the double-pass scheme. The preamplifiers should be designed such that fluctuations in the oscillator pulse energy can be smoothed out. Saturation should therefore already be partially achieved in the second amplifier during the second pass. Output energies of up to 5 Joules can then easily be obtained.

Main Amplifiers. In the previous section it was shown that for the maximum stored inversion energy density of 6.5 J/cm^2, permitted by the maximum argon buffer gas pressure of 6 bar for a small-signal amplification of 100 (a value typical of main amplifiers also), an extraction efficiency of about 60% will be obtained for input energy densities higher than 1.6 J/cm^2. This fact raises the question whether the achievement of a high extraction efficiency has to be the main goal in designing an iodine laser system. An input energy density of 1.6 J/cm^2 will only allow an energy amplification factor of 2.2 and 3.75 to be achieved at the maximum output energy densities of 3.5 and 6 J/cm^2, respectively. Thus the number of amplifiers for a desired chain output can be too large, and the relation of cost to output energy will then be unfavourable. It is therefore more economical to operate the amplifiers with pulses having lower input energy densities at the cost of a lower extraction efficiency. The losses will then be more than compensated by the saving in capital costs for the construction of amplifiers and their auxiliary equipment. In addition, benefits are to be expected from the improved reliability of the system and the reduced maintenance effort.

Another argument for minimizing the number of amplifiers is based on the fact that a larger number of amplifiers will lead to higher pulse energy absorption losses in saturable absorbers or Pockels cells installed for the decoupling of adjacent amplifiers and for keeping the net small-signal amplification of the chain at a level such that the prepulse energy does not exceed a value prescribed by laser plasma experiments. The higher gain originating from the higher extraction efficiency of amplifiers with low energy amplification factors may then be more than compensated by the losses in the decoupling elements.

To find an optimum configuration for the main amplifier chain, an energy balance for minimizing the electrical pumping energy E_{el} stored in the capacitor bank at a given output energy has to be made. According to the (5.5, 7, 9) this electric energy is determined by the following relation:

$$E_{el} = \frac{E_{out} - E_{in}}{KP\eta_{ex}\eta_{el}} \quad . \tag{5.11}$$

Introducing an energy amplification factor $A_i = (E_{out})_i/(E_{in})_i$, for the ith amplifier, (5.11) reads

$$(E_{el})_i = \frac{(E_{out})_i}{K_iP_i(\eta_{ex})_i(\eta_{el})_i}\,(1 - 1/A_i) \quad . \tag{5.12}$$

When the energy transmission factor $L_i = (E_{in})_i/(E_{out})_{i-1}$ between two adjacent amplifiers (i-1) and i is known, the total electric energy supply $(E_{el})_{tot}$ for the amplifier chain can be calculated provided that the output energy $(E_{out})_{EA}$ of the end amplifier is defined and the output energy of the preamplifier $(E_{out})_{PA}$ fed into the chain is given. Both values determine the total energy amplification factor $(LA)_{tot}$ of a chain of n main amplifiers

$$(LA)_{tot} = \frac{(E_{out})_{EA}}{(E_{out})_{PA}} = \prod_{j=1}^{n} L_jA_j \quad . \tag{5.13}$$

Summing up all contributions to the electric pumping energy of the chain one obtains

$$(E_{el})_{tot} = \sum_{i=1}^{n} \frac{(E_{out})_{PA}\prod_{j=1}^{i} L_jA_j}{K_iP_i(\eta_{ex})_i(\eta_{el})_i}\,(1 - 1/A_i) \quad . \tag{5.14}$$

This equation allows the determination of the optimal chain configuration, which is defined by the minimum of the total electrical pumping energy of the main amplifier chain for a sufficiently small number of amplifiers.

In optimizing the amplifier chain, one needs to start with the end amplifier. Its effective diameter d_{eff} is defined by (5.1) when the output energy $(E_{out})_{EA}$ and the maximum loading of the output window e_m are specified. First of all, the input energy density e_{in}, has to be chosen such that at a sufficiently high value of the energy amplification factor A_i and a reasonably high value of the extraction efficiency ($\eta_{ex} \geqq 50\%$) is provided. The value of e_{in} enables η_{ex} to be determined by an iterative process (with at most two steps), when the dependence of η_{ex} on e_{in} is given for various stored energy densities at a prescribed small-signal amplification. In the first step, the value of η_{ex} can be estimated at the evaluated e_{in} value from the set of $\eta_{ex} = f(e_{in}, e_{st}, A_{ss})$ curves (Fig. 5.1). Then e_{st} can be approximated according to the relation $e_{st} = (e_{out} - e_{in})/\eta_{ex}$ This e_{st} value allows the second approximation of the η_{ex} and e_{st} values. Finally it has to be determined whether the limitations for the buffer gas pressure $p = f(e_{st}, A_{ss})$ will not be violated by the evaluated e_{st} value (Fig. 3.3). The value of $(\eta_{el})_i$ can be calculated with the (5.2, 3, 4, 6) at the given values of the pumping time T_p, the beam divergence and the speed of the shock wave a_s. K_i and P_i are defined by the (5.6, 7).

The product $(E_{in})_i L_i$ (L-transmission factor) now determines the output energy of the preceeding amplifier. Its specifications can be calculated by the method just described. Using an empirical process, the energy amplification factors A_i of all the individual main amplifiers of the chain can now be chosen such that at the specified values of $(E_{out})_{EA}/ (E_{out})_{PA}$ together with the given energy transmission factors L_i, (5.13) is satisfied with minimized electrical pumping energy.

In Fig. 5.3 the dependence of the total electric pumping energy on the energy amplification factor A_{EA} of the end amplifier is shown for an amplifier chain, which amplifies the 5 J output energy from the preamplifier chain to a level of 500 J. Each main amplifier has a small-signal amplification of 100, the energy transmission factors L_i being always 0.7, the ratio $K = F_{eff}/F_{tot}$ ranging between $0.5 \leqq K \leqq 0.8$ and $P \cong (E_{st})_{Tp}/(E_{st})_{tot}$ has a value of 0.75 for diameters less than 20 cm and for larger diameters a value of 0.8. The limiting parameter in this analysis is the maximum energy density loading of the output windows. Its value is fixed at e_m = 3.5 J/cm^2 (for dielectric AR coating) and 6 J/cm^2 (for graded index surfaces) respectively. For the chain configurations calculated, the stored

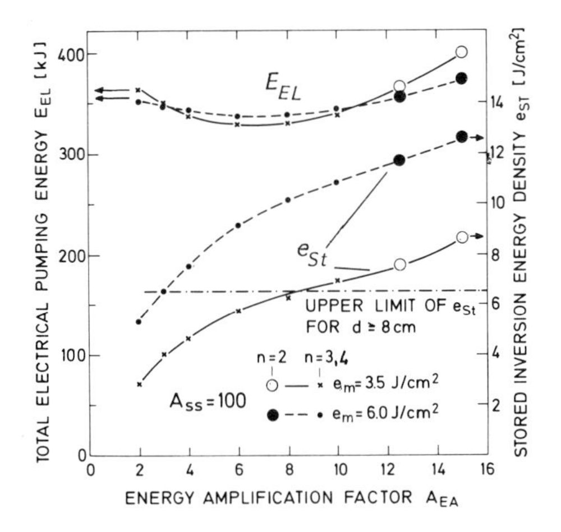

Fig. 5.3. Total electrical pumping energy of the main amplifiers (left ordinate) and stored inversion energy density of the end amplifier (right ordinate) vs energy amplification factor A_{EA} of the end amplifier of a chain with an output energy of 500 J (output energy densities: 3.5 and 6.0 J/cm^2)

inversion energy density of the end amplifier is also plotted versus the energy amplification factor A_{EA}.

The performance of the chain was calculated for n = 2, 3 and 4 main amplifiers. The electric pumping energy for the 4 amplifier chain is not specified in Fig. 5.3 because these values are only a few per cent smaller than those calculated for a n = 3 chain. The saving in the capacitor bank will therefore not compensate the greater effort required for the construction of the fourth amplifier and its auxiliary equipment. Since a fixed energy amplification factor of the output amplifier allows in a n = 3 chain various combinations of the energy amplification factors of the first and second main amplifiers, only the minimum values for $(E_{el})_{tot}$ have been plotted in Fig. 5.3.

Both curves show a minimum in the A_{EA}-value range between 6 and 8. This is due to the fact that for large amplification factors ($A_{EA} \geqq 8$) the input energy density of the end amplifier is correspondingly reduced and thus, according to the curves of Fig. 5.1, the extraction efficiency η_{ex} has a smaller value. The same is true for small amplification factors ($A_{EA} \leqq 6$) when energy amplification factors of the first and second amplifiers are high. Because of the smaller sizes of these amplifiers, the increase of $(E_{el})_{tot}$ is here less pronounced than in the case of the much larger end amplifier. The weaker increase of $(E_{el})_{tot}$ for the curve e_m = 6 J/cm^2 in these regions is due to the fact that here e_{in} is still much closer to the saturation energy density, and thus the decrease in η_{ex} is less strong than for the curve e_m = 3.5 J/cm^2.

In the region $4 \leqq A_{EA} \leqq 10$, where the input energy density for all amplifiers is closest to the saturation energy density, the amplifiers possessing $e_m = 6\ J/cm^2$ require the higher electric pumping energy, although these amplifiers have higher input energy densities and thus higher extraction efficiencies η_{ex}. This discrepancy is explained by the fact that the $e_m = 6\ J/cm^2$ amplifiers have smaller amplifier diameters ($d_{eff} = 10$ cm for the end amplifier) and therefore the reduction of the ratio $K = F_{eff}/F_{tot}$ is a stronger factor than the increase of η_{ex}. For a chain whose end amplifier has an effective diameter $d_{eff} > 20$ cm the trend reverses, because the increase in η_{ex} will be stronger than the reduction of K.

For amplifiers with diameters $d > 8$ cm and a maximum small signal amplification $A_{ss} \cong 100$, the upper limit for the stored inversion energy density is $e_{st} \leqq 6.5\ J/cm^2$ because of the proposed buffer gas pressure restrictions ($p_{Ar} \leqq 6$ bar). According to Fig. 5.3 amplifiers with an output energy density of $e_m = 6\ J/cm^2$ can therefore only be operated at energy amplification factors smaller than 3, and those with $e_m = 3.5\ J/cm^2$ at energy amplification factors of up to 8.

With decreasing energy amplification factors, the stored inversion energy density and thus also the buffer gas pressure necessary to keep the small-signal amplification at the prescribed level decreases. The length of the end amplifier, the required electric pumping energy, and the effort for handling the buffer gas pressure therefore also decrease. For these reasons the smallest energy amplification factor would be the cheapest solution for the end amplifier, and also the most suitable for shifting the threshold for the occurence of self-focusing effects to shorter pulse lengths. This is because lower buffer gas pressures permit thinner amplifier windows, especially for the large diameter amplifiers. As the output windows in an iodine laser make a significant contribution to the value of the B integral, their thickness should therefore be minimized. The requirement of shifting the region for the occurrence of self-focusing effects to pulse lengths as short as possible is also an important aspect in designing an amplifier chain. This calls for fewer windows and hence fewer amplifiers.

In spite of these arguments, the smallest energy amplification factor of the end amplifier is not the optimal solution for the chain. This is because the requirements placed upon the first and second amplifier increase with a decreasing amplification factor of the end amplifier. Optimization of the two opposing trends leads to the determination of a minimum in the construction costs of the chain. Because the costs of the end amplifier represent the larger portion of the total costs of the chain, the minimum of the construction costs of the chain will be positioned at an A_{EA} value smaller than the value characterizing the minimum of $(E_{el})_{tot}$. Taking into account cost, beam quality, and also technical considerations, the most suitable design for the main amplifier chain with an output energy density of e_m = 3.5 J/cm^2 is expected to be at an energy amplification factor of about 4 for the end amplifier.

For a chain with amplifier output energy densities of 6 J/cm^2, only an end amplifier with an energy amplification factor of 3 will not violate the restrictions for the buffer gas pressure. Although smaller amplification factors are still feasible for this amplifier, they cannot be realized because they require excessively high buffer gas pressure in the first and second amplifiers.

5.1.3 The Configuration of a 500 J Amplifier Chain

The characteristics of a complete iodine laser chain capable of delivering an output energy of 500 J are shown in Fig. 5.4. The performance of this chain is illustrated in Fig. 5.5 by plotting the amplifier input and output energies versus the stored inversion energy. Two preamplifiers, of which the second is operated in the double-pass scheme, provide the energy to initiate saturation of the first main amplifier. The energy amplification factors of the three main amplifiers are 10, 6, and 4. The relevant data of all the amplifiers are specified in the insert of Fig. 5.5. Two Pockels

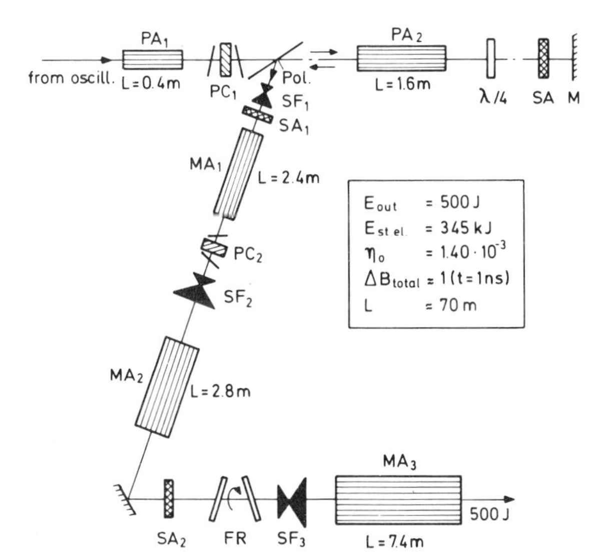

Fig. 5.4. Scheme of an iodine laser chain with an output energy of 500 J

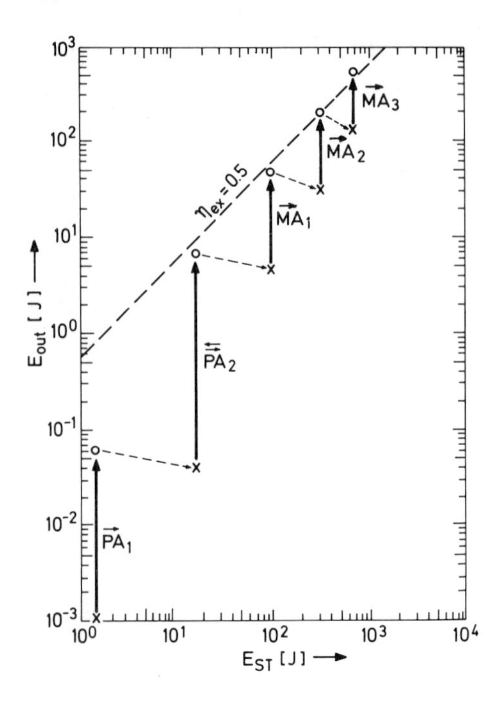

L = 0.7	$\overrightarrow{PA}_1$	$\overleftrightarrow{PA}_2$	$\overrightarrow{MA}_1$	$\overrightarrow{MA}_2$	$\overrightarrow{MA}_3$
A_{ss}	100	200	100	100	100
A_i	50	170	10	6	4
η_{ex}	0.18	0.37	0.44	0.51	0.56
e_{St} [J/cm^2]	2.1	6.7	7.2	5.7	4.7
p_{Ar} [bar]	0.85	3.8	7.4	6.0	5.3
e_{out} [J/cm^2]	0.26	2.4	3.5	3.5	3.5
E_{el} [kJ]	1.0	8.8	35	110	190
d_{eff} [cm]	0.5	1.8	4.0	8.1	13.5

Fig. 5.5. Amplifier input and output energies vs stored inversion energy of a laser system with an output energy of 500 J

cells and two saturable absorbers placed between the amplifiers are used for optical isolation of adjacent amplifiers and for prepulse suppression. A Faraday rotator, located between the second and third main amplifiers, serves to protect the system from light retro-reflected from the target. In addition, spatial filters designed to achieve image relaying and beam expansion are installed. All these elements lead to an energy transmission factor between adjacent amplifiers having a value of approximately $L_i = 0.7$.

The amplifier chain is designed such that the extraction efficiency increases along the chain and achieves its maximum value of 56% in the end amplifier. With a total electric pumping energy of 345 kJ, the overall laser efficiency is 0.14%.

The discussion in the previous sections has dealt primarily with energy considerations for pulse lengths restricted to 1 ns. Laser plasma experiments require, however, pulses with lengths ranging from the subnanosecond to the several nanosecond region. Since a substantial pulse shortening and steepening takes place in a saturated amplifier chain (see Sect. 3.3.4), a correspondingly longer input pulse has to be injected into the amplifier chain to obtain the desired output pulse length. The relation between the input and the output pulse lengths can be calculated with the computer simulation code given in Sect. 3.3.4.

The layout of the amplifier chain described in Fig. 5.4 is such that the optical beam loading will not exceed the maximum output energy density e_m permitted by the damage threhold of AR coatings for pulse lengths of 1 ns. At this pulse length, the value of the B integral at the exit of the output amplifier is approximately equal to unity. This value therefore does not require the use of a spatial filter in order to maintain a satisfactory beam homogeneity. When pulses with lengths exceeding 1 ns are propagated, the output energy of the laser can be increased according to the damage threshold-pulse width relation reported in [5.2]. Since with increasing pulse length the damage threshold has a weaker dependence on the pulse length than the B integral the laser performance remains always fluence limited.

Pulses with lengths in the subnanosecond region will lead to damage problems at the desired output energy of 500 J. The output energy therefore has to be correspondingly reduced. The dependence of the damage threshold on the pulse length is in this region not yet definitely established. Measurements indicate that the relation between pulse width and damage threshold is nearly the same as for pulses with lengths exceeding 1 ns. For pulse lengths shorter than 500 ns properly staged spatial filters are required to control small scale self-focusing. Down to pulse duration of about 50 ps the system design, however, still remains fluence limited because the increasing of the B integral even for an amplifier working primarily in the saturation regime is not larger than 2.

In concluding this section it can be stated that the first-order scaling laws and guide lines for the design of an amplifier chain will not yield a laser system with the highest efficiency. Limitations arising from the need to obtain an almost homogeneous inversion profile do not allow the achievement of maximum pumping efficiency, and the maximum value of the extraction efficiency cannot be obtained either. This situation arises because the energy amplification factor per amplifier would otherwise be too small and hence the necessary number of amplifiers too large. The overall cost for components and their subsequent maintenance would then not be minimized, and the larger number of components reqired for amplifier isolation would reduce overall system efficiency.

The design criteria outlined here will yield, with the limitations imposed by the maximum permissible buffer gas pressure and by the damage threshold of components, a laser system with minimum costs, using current technology and having an acceptable efficiency. It thus represents a reasonable compromise in meeting the economical and operational requirements for an iodine laser system determined for laser fusion experiments.

5.2 Active Laser Components

The active components of the iodine laser, the oscillator and the amplifiers, have features not shared by other high-power lasers. In particular, these special characteristics include the need for replacing and regenerating the laser medium after each firing of the laser and a special optical pumping technology.

5.2.1 Laser Tubes and Laser Medium Handling

The basic setup of the oscillator and the amplifiers consists of cylindrical quartz tubes containing the laser medium, and linear flashlamps with reflectors surrounding them. The quartz wall material of the laser tubes should be chosen such that transmission of pumplight with a wavelength shorter than 200 nm is blocked, otherwise the efficiency of the pumping process may be reduced by carbon deposits on the laser tube walls arising from photolysis of the laser medium [5.3]. Also the predominant production of ground state iodine, when the pumping spectrum covers the VUV region at 155 to 175 nm, will decrease the inversion [5.4].

The most common alkyliodides used for the active medium are either iso- or n-perfluoropropyl iodide (C_3F_7I). In amplifiers employing a closed cycle laser medium regeneration system [5.5] i-C_3F_7I is to be preferred for practical reasons, since it requires less cooling for the same pressure. Highly purified liquid C_3F_7I (both iso and n) is commercially available. However, before it is used as a laser medium, dissolved gaseous compounds, such as oxygen, have to be removed by multiple fractional destillation. The C_3F_7I pressure p_{RI} in the laser tube depends on its diameter d. For U-shaped reflectors it is given by the relation $p_{RI}d$ = 200 mbar cm (Sect. 3.2.3).

After a firing of the laser, the active medium does not completely regenerate. As a consequence the partial pressure of the C_3F_7I is reduced and molecular iodine, a strong quencher of excited iodine atoms, is formed. It is therefore necessary to regenerate the laser medium of the oscillator and the amplifiers after each shot. This can be accomplished by an automatic closed cyle regeneration system [5.5]. It purifies the laser gas by condensing the molecular iodine and restores the correct C_3F_7I pressure by passing the gas through a vessel where stored liquid C_3F_7I is cooled to a temperature at which its vapour pressure corresponds to the required partial pressure in the laser tubes. For laser operation the temperatures of the storage vessels for the different laser tube cross sections range from -10° to about -50°C, according to the vapour pressure to temperature relation given for i-C_3F_7I in Fig. 5.6. The regeneration time for the laser medium depends on the cooled surface area in the C_3F_7I storage vessel. In present systems it ranges from 1 to 10 min.

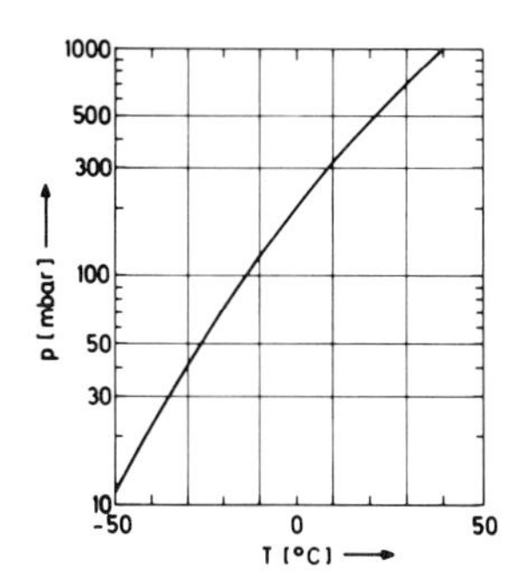

Fig. 5.6. Vapour pressure of i-C_3F_7I vs temperature

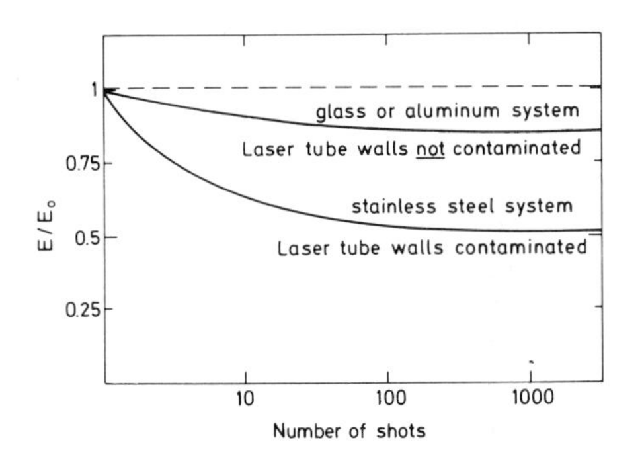

Fig. 5.7. Normalized output energy as a function of the shot number for a glass or aluminium and a stainless steel regeneration system

A further closed cycle regeneration system, developed by BAKER and KING [5.6] is particularly well suited for high repetition rate oscillators or small iodine laser amplifiers. Systems of this type utilize thermally driven gas flow for replenishment. The flow is produced by thermal evaporation from a heated vessel and subsequent condensation at the desired cold temperature at which the required vapour pressure of C_3F_7I is obtained. When using condensable heavy fluorocarbons as a buffer gas, the amplification properties of the laser medium can be modified in a certain range.

For the case that laser medium will be exchanged after each shot, GAVRILINA et al. [5.7] have developed a method for recyling the laser medium when SF_6 is used as a buffer gas. Its operation is based upon freezing out the exhausted laser medium and subsequent separation of the purified C_3F_7I and SF_6 by fractional distillation.

In iodine laser amplifiers even with a regeneration of the laser medium after each shot a gradual decrease of the stored inversion energy with increasing shot number can be observed. It may result in an energy loss of up to 50% for a newly assembled system within the first 50 to 100 shots (Fig. 5.7).

The reasons for this energy decline are the following. A minor contribution to the lowering of the amplifier efficiency is caused by UV light induced formation of colour centres (solarization) within the volume of both the quartz flashlamps and the laser tubes. It reduces the transmission in the near UV region of the spectrum (up to 15%) and saturates at a level of about hundred shots. This effect is particularly noticable with quartz glasses which absorb in the region of 200-230 nm. Ultrapure quartz (such as suprasil) shows only little solarization.

A more severe degradation of the pumping efficiency is sometimes caused by the formation of pumplight absorping layers on the inner walls of the quartz laser tube. Several kinds of such layers have been observed in iodine lasers.

In a laser medium regeneration system containing metal components, molecular iodine formed after photolysis reacts slowly with the metal to form metal iodides. Especially susceptible are parts made from copper, brass, zinc or nickel. Stainless steel is also attacked by I_2. Metal iodide particles are then swept around in the system by the gas flow and deposit as a dark powder on the laser tube, thereby reducing the efficiency of the pumping process. It has been found, however, that deposition of metal iodides and the resulting energy losses can be avoided by using a laser medium regeneration system containing only glass and aluminum components.

A darkening of the tube walls by carbon deposits is frequently observed in iodine lasers. PADRICK and PALMER [5.3] attributed the formation of these deposits to photolysis of $i\text{-}C_3F_7I$ (or other parent compounds) caused by UV irradiation at wavelengths below 200 nm. They found that carbon deposition can be avoided by the use of titanium-doped quartz for the laser tube. This quartz transmits well in the laser pump band but is opaque at wavelengths below 200 nm.

A frequent source of carbon deposits is caused by hydrocarbons absorbed onto the inner walls of the laser tube. Mineral oils, for example, react with photolysis products to form a dark layer of carbon in the UV-illuminated region of an amplifier. The mechanism is probably hydrogen extraction by the free radical of the alkyl iodide.

Hydrocarbon contamination of the laser tube wall can occur with forepump oil or with lubricating oils from the circulation pump. Additional sources of contamination may arise from the cleaning procedure of the laser tube prior to assembly or the UV-induced decomposition of vacuum grease.

To avoid the formation of such absorbing carbon layers care has to be taken in the design and assembly of a system. Forepumps should be baffled with oil filters and liquid nitrogen traps. In the circulation system, membrane pumps provide an oil-free gas flow. As little vacuum grease as possible should be applied to all vacuum joints. A further precautionary measure is the use of hydrocarbon-free oils and greases. Fully fluorinated oil, for example, is extremely stable and will not be decomposed by UV irradiation in the presence of photolysis products of the alkyl iodide.

It was experimentally proven that except for the relatively small energy decline caused by the formation of colour centers in the quartz material, all the other losses can be avoided by a suitable system design and assembly. This means that the system performance can be maintained for hundreds of shots with a reduction $\leq 15\%$.

When using a laser with a closed cycle laser medium regeneration system the entire system containing the laser medium (tubes, storage vessels for the alkyliodide etc.) have to be vacuum tight in order to avoid quenching of excited iodine atoms by atmospheric impurities (Sect. 2.3.5). In particular, oxygen is a very strong quencher and the partial pressure of O_2 should therefore be kept below a level of 10^{-1} mbar for laser tubes with flashlamp pumping times of the order of 10 μs (scaling inversely proportional to the pumping time). The leak rate of the amplifier and the associated regeneration system should not exceed values in the range from 10^{-2} to 10^{-6} mbar l/s (decreasing with decreasing volumes). When the alkyl iodide has been consumed, the storage vessel of the regeneration system should be evacuated to a pressure of approximately 10^{-3} mbar before it can be replenished. This is to assure that all the contaminants (I_2, O_2) are removed.

5.2.2 Optical Pumping System

The oscillator and the amplifiers are pumped by flashlamps made from quartz tubes. They are filled with xenon at a pressure of 40 mbar. Experiments have demonstrated that this pressure provides the maximum efficiency of 7% to 9% for converting electric energy into UV radiation lying in the pump band of the alkyl iodide (Sect. 2.2.2). The maximum pumping time scales with increasing tube diameter as shown in Sect. 4.2.1 Eq. (4.6). For the systems now in use it covers the region from 1.5 to 12 μs. The dimensions of the flashlamps of present systems are as follows: Their internal diameters range from 8 to 25 mm, whereas their lengths are between 40 and 100 cm. Two types of lamps are in use: the sealed commercial and the operator-refillable flashlamps. Both types of lamps have to be replaced after 1000 to 3000 shots because an increasing number of microcracks in the quartz walls primarily in the region of the electrodes raises the probability of lamp explosion. For the sealed flashlamps, in addition, the decreasing UV yield with increasing shot number calls for a lamp replacement. This decrease is due to the increasing impurity level in the xenon gas, thus lowering the electron temperature. In refillable flashlamps this effect can be avoided by renewing the xenon gas after a 20 to 30 shot cycle. These flashlamps need a refilling system and consume xenon. This disadvantage is, however, compensated by the fact that the installation of costly fault-sensing equipment, necessary in large laser systems to avoid flashlamp explosion problems caused by flashlamp leakage, is not required. The state of such flashlamps is controlled by measuring the pressure in the central refilling system.

The replacement intervals of the flashlamps can be greatly prolonged if the loading of the lamps is decreased slightly or by applying a simmer current [5.8]. Likewise a symmetrizing of the electric field distribution in the flashlamp prior to their ignition will remarkably prolong their lifetimes. Due to this symmetrizing the resulting current distribution in the flashlamp is much more homogeneous and the current no longer flows preferentially along the quartz wall. Thus a reduction of thermal wall loading and subsequent ablation will result. The symmetric electric field distribution can be produced by placing one or two wires at suitable locations between the flashlamp and the laser quartz tube in the case in which the flashlamp reflector is used for the flashlamp return current path [5.9]. These wires are connected to the reflector at one end only so that they have the same potential as the reflector. First tests of this geometry with the iodine laser indicate that the lifetimes of the flashlamps were approximately doubled.

Transparency measurements of the flashlamps revealed that the xenon plasma is optically dense to the radiation overlapping the alkyliodide pumping band. This fact has to be taken into account when optimizing the reflector geometry. The reflectors for the flashlamps are preferably made of electropolished pure aluminium sheets (99.99% Al). Because of the presence of thin Al_2O_3 layers, their reflectivity at λ = 280 nm is only 70%

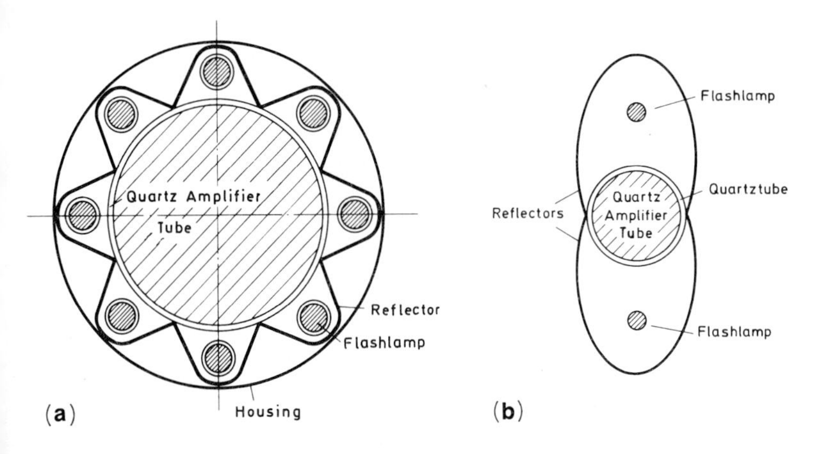

Fig. 5.8a,b. Cross-section of amplifiers with U-shaped (a) and elliptic (b) reflectors

or less. In general, U-shaped reflectors (Fig. 5.8.a) are employed. With these reflectors a relatively large fraction of the pumplight emitted in the outward direction and then reflected into the flashlamp is absorbed in the optically thick xenon plasma. This fraction decreases, however, with increasing opening angle of the reflectors when the interlamp spacing is enlarged. The most effective pumplight coupling will, however, be obtained by using an elliptic reflector geometry arranged in such a way that the flashlamp is positioned in one focus, whereas the other focus coincides with the axis of the amplifier (Fig. 5.8b). The elliptic reflector geometry has, in addition, the advantage of improving the inversion profile and thus allowing a higher C_3F_7I pressure and hence better pumplight absorption. This reflector arrangement is, however, not suitable for large aperture amplifiers because they require excessive space and are then too costly. In any case a cost-benefit analysis should be made before applying them.

For generating adequate quantities of UV light, low inductance capacitor banks with short pump pulse durations have to be installed. For the oscillator and the amplifiers, the duration of a discharge half-cycle should be in the microsecond range. This requirement calls for low inductance capacitors, transmission lines, spark gaps and flashlamp installations. In addition, to ensure efficient and rapid energy coupling into the flashlamps and to stress the capacitors as little as possible, the circuit inductance and resistance have to be adequately matched to prevent voltage reversals higher than 25%. Under these conditions approximately 70% of the electrical energy stored in the capacitor bank is released during the first half-cycle.

The capacitor banks of the laser system should preferably be built in a module system. For effective and low-inductance energy storage, the capacitor charging voltage should be in the range of 40 kV. It has already been demonstrated that up to four flashlamps can be operated in parallel in one circuit switched by one spark gap with a jitter less than 0.1 μs and a voltage reversal not higher than 20% [5.10].

5.2.3 Oscillator

The different methods of generating short pulses have already been described in Sect. 3.1. Since the method presently preferred is active mode-locking, the following considerations will be restricted to this technique.

In addition to achieving reliable and reproducible operation, a pulse generating system should be capable of producing pulses with energies of at least 1 mJ (this energy is needed for reliable operation employing a laser-triggered spark gap). Such a system should allow the variation of the pulse length from the subnanosecond to the nanosecond region, and it should provide a diffraction-limited beam. Furthermore a shot-to-shot directional beam stability of less than 20 μrad and a shot rate of at least one shot every 2 min are desirable.

These requirements can be met by an acousto-optically mode-locked oscillator. For the generation of pulses with diffraction limited beam quality, stable and unstable resonator configurations can be used. Because of its high insensitivity to misalignment semiconfocal cavity configurations operated in the TEM_{00} are usually preferred. The cavity length at the ordinary modulator frequencies of 30 to 50 MHz ranges from 150 to 250 cm. To maintain consistant alignment of the beam, the cavity mirrors have to be mounted on a stable granite bench or on Invar rails, both isolated from floor vibrations. In addition, the resonator cavity length must be precisely matched to the modulator frequency to maintain reliable operation, and the oscillator should be situated in a temperature controlled environment with a temperature stability of better than ± 1°C.

The length of the quartz tube containing the laser medium usually ranges from 50 to 100 cm, with an inner diameter of up to 1 cm. According to the $p_{RI}d$ = 200 mbar cm relation the pressure of the alkyliodide is then 200 mbar.

The oscillator should be pumped with an electrical energy of about 1 kJ to obtain a pulse energy of a single pulse in the range of 1 mJ. As the beam quality of the oscillator output pulses may be impaired by shock waves or by optical inhomogeneities caused by non-uniform heating of the laser medium (Sect. 4.2.1), the pumping time should be as short as possible thus requiring a discharge circuit with a duration of a half-cycle no longer than 2 μs.

As already described in Sect. 2.1.5, the magnetic field caused by the flashlamp currents will split the hyperfine levels of the laser transition differently. As a consequence, the σ values of the individual laser transitions will be differently reduced, those for the lines of the 3-4 transition more strongly than those for the lines of the 2-2 transition. Therefore, at low buffer gas pressures, the pulse emitted from the oscillator will only contain the spectrum of the 2-2 transition at a magnetic field strength of about 500 A/cm. In addition, strong magnetic fields will polarize the emitted radiation.

Since for laser operation the line of the 3-4 transition is favoured, and uncontrollable polarization should be avoided, the magnetic field in the mode volume should be kept below a value of 100 A/cm. This can be achieved by arranging the flashlamps symmetrically at a sufficiently large distance around the laser tube, with their currents flowing in parallel. In this case the contributions of the different flashlamps will effectively compensate each other in the mode volume.

According to the Siegman-Kuizenga theory [5.11], pulses with durations in the range from 0.2 ns to about 1.5 ns can be generated in an actively mode-locked oscillator. The bandwidth of the laser transition then has to be adjusted between 25 and 2 GHz, and a modulation index between 1.0 and 1.5 at a modulator frequency in the range from 30 to 50 MHz should be obtained [see (3.1)].

The bandwidth for the required pulse length will be adjusted by appropriate broadening on the laser transition with argon or SF_6 as a buffer gas (see Fig. 3.2). To obtain the above specified minimum pulse length the buffer gas pressure has to be raised to a value of 8 bar.

The modulation index sufficiently high for reproducible generation of short pulses will be provided when a fused silica modulator is powered in pulsed operation (pulse lengths 1 ms) by a pulse at the required frequency with a power of about 20 to 50 W. A modulation index of up to 1.5 can then be obtained [5.12]. As the resonance frequency of the mode locker is temperature dependent, its temperature has to be stabilized within a limit of ± 0.2°C.

5.2.4 Amplifiers

The basic geometry for the construction of the amplifiers is the same as for the oscillators: A quartz tube containing the laser medium surrounded by linear flashlamps and their reflectors oriented parallel to the laser tube axis. Since for amplifiers different from the oscillator, the full area free from disturbances caused by the flashlamp-induced shock waves must be available for the pulse amplificaton, it is necessary to eliminate the focusing of the pump light reflected from the cylindrical surface of the opposing quartz wall (caustic effect). Otherwise excessive inversion densities will arise, producing undesirable hot spots in the output beam. These internal reflections can be effectively controlled by either sand-blasting or etching the internal walls such that an optically diffuse surface is obtained. This, however, also reduces the pumping efficiency by approximately 10%.

The input and output windows of the amplifiers must be of high optical quality to permit the maximum amplifier radiance to be achieved. To suppress parasitic oscillations, the windows can be oriented nearly normal to the tube axis when supplied with anti-reflective surfaces or have to be positioned at Brewester's angle when bare surfaces are used. Brewster windows, however, give a larger contribution to the B integral because of their inclination and their significantly larger thickness, and, in addition, they impair the system alignment due to beam offset effects when the optical alignment is, for example, carried out with a HeNe laser. Thus windows oriented nearly perpendicular to the amplifier axis are preferred. The AR coatings of these windows can be provided as shown in Sect. 5.3.2 by dielectric coatings (median damage threshold at $\tau_p = 1$ ns, $e_d \leqq 8$ J/cm^2) or graded index surfaces (damage threshold at $\tau_p = 1$ ns, $e_d \cong 12$ J/cm^2).

Because the pressures of the alkyl iodide and the buffer gas of the individual amplifiers differ, each amplifier has to be equipped with its own regeneration system for the laser medium. The maximum buffer gas pressure in large aperture main amplifiers is up to 6 bar. To preserve the optical quality of the laser beam at this pressure the thickness of the amplifier windows has to be chosen such that the windows will not bend.

To store the inversion energy, the value of the small signal amplification in an amplifier has to be below the threshold for internal and external parasitic oscillations. For amplifiers incorporated into a laser system this value is up to a few hundred (Sect. 5.1.2). The small-signal amplification in an amplifier can easily be adjusted to a value below this threshold by pressure broadening of the laser transition. For the inversion densities attainable in amplifiers, σ values in the range from 8×10^{-19} to 1×10^{-19} cm^2 have to be selected. These values can be provided by argon or SF_6 pressures from 0.5 to 6 bar. The dimensions of the amplifier tubes are determined by the scaling laws given in Sect. 3.2 and by the design criteria outlined in Sect. 5.1.1.

The preamplifiers (whose maximum dimensions will not exceed an inner tube diameter of 3.5 cm) are usually assembled from one or two sections with an active length of about 1 m. They are pumped by two to four flashlamps per section with internal diameters of up to 12 mm. For effective pumplight coupling elliptic reflectors can be employed. The electric energy of their capacitor banks ranges from 1 to 10 kJ at a duration of the discharge half-cycle in the range of 2 to 4 μs. To restrict the refraction losses caused by the shock waves, the stored energy in the amplifiers needs to be extracted after a pumping duration of from 5 to 7 μs. The partial pressure of the alkyl iodide lies between 60 and 100 mbar, and that of the buffer gas between 0.5 and 3.5 bar when argon or SF_6 is used.

It is convenient to assemble a main amplifier from individual sections with an active length of 1 to 1.5 m. With external flashlamp pumping each section is composed of a quartz tube, a metal housing as a supporting structure, and the flashlamps with their reflectors mounted between the quartz tube and the housing.

The number of sections depends, according to (5.2,3), on the amplifier diameter. The upper bound for the amplifier diameter is only subjected to practical limitations. A beam diameter of 50 cm seems to be a reasonable upper limit for external flashlamp pumping since otherwise the required C_3F_7I pressure and hence the stored inversion density (per cm^3) becomes too low. These amplifiers will be pumped by flashlamps with internal diameters of up to a few cm.

Because of cost and space considerations in main amplifiers, elliptic reflectors can no longer be used. Instead U-shaped reflectors should be employed (Fig. 5.8a). The stored electrical energy of their capacitor banks ranges for large aperture amplifiers up into the MJ range. The duration of the discharge half-cycle ranges from 4 to 12 μs, and the stored inversion energy in the amplifiers has to be extracted after a pumping time of 7 to 15 μs. The partial pressure of the alkyl iodide is within the values of 5 to 50 mbar when external flashlamp pumping is used. The argon or SF_6 pressure is up to 6 bar.

According to (5.2,3) the length of an amplifier increases linearly with the amplifier diameter when with external flashlamp pumping the specific inversion density u is held constant. The length of amplifiers can, however, be reduced by mounting additional flashlamps inside the laser medium. In this case the value of the specific inversion density will be raised and, in addition, the pumplight can be deposited at a higher alkyl iodide pressure while maintaining still an adequate inversion homogeneity. This additional internal pumping will also increase the pumping efficiency by 10% to 20% because of the better pumplight coupling. However, flashlamps in contact with the active medium create optical inhomogeneities which disturb the optical quality of the laser beam. They also obscure portions of the amplifier aperture. In addition, the inside lamps would be difficult to install electrically and would require a separate cooling system. These disadvantages need to be weighed against the advantages associated with internal lamps, namely, shorter amplifier lengths and higher pumping efficiencies.

Experience has shown that the heat released by the flashlamps pumping the laser medium leads to a vertical temperature gradient (Sect. 4.3.1) and hence to a vertical refractive index gradient. This in turn induces disturbances of the directional stability of the laser beam. To prevent the formation of these gradients, the quartz tubes of the main and also those of the preamplifiers have to be cooled. For this purpose preferably a closed loop He gas cooling system should be used. It requires less effort than a water cooling system and guarantees an effective heat exchange due to the favourable heat transport characteristics of helium. An open air cooling system tends to be disadvantageous because it gradually impairs the reflectivity of the flashlamp reflectors by dust deposition, and, in addition, the ozone formed during the firing of the flashlamps will partially absorb the pump light and may attack the surface of the aluminium reflectors.

5.3 Passive Components of the Laser System

In an amplifier chain several passive elements have to be incorporated into the laser chain for selection of the pulse to be amplified, expansion of the beam cross-section, prepulse suppression and optical isolation of the amplifiers, and protection of sensitive laser components against damage by laser light retro-reflected from the target. Further equipment is necessary for laser alignment and control of laser operation.

5.3.1 Pulse Selection System

To gate out the pulse to be amplified from the mode-locked pulse train of the oscillator, a pulse selection system, consisting of Pockels cells with their polarizers and the electrical system for switching the Pockels cells, has to be used. For satisfactory suppression of the prepulse energy caused by leakage of the oscillator pulse train through the closed pulse selection system, two or three Pockels cells have to be installed in series, otherwise a sufficiently high contrast ratio cannot be achieved. KD*P crystals have to be used in the Pockels cells to provide a high transmission of the laser radiation

The rectangular high-voltage pulse of 8 to 10 kV with a length corresponding to the oscillator round trip time (i.e. 16 ns for a 30 MHz modulator frequency) for driving the Pockels cells can be generated by a pulse forming network of a properly chosen cable and initiated by a laser triggered spark gap. For reliable operation, the jitter in the breakdown of the spark gap should not be higher than 2-3 ns, but because of the statistical nature of the electrical breakdown phenomena in the laser-triggered spark gaps, for 1 mJ oscillator pulses the jitter may be as great as 8 ns, decreasing with increasing pulse energy. Due to this relatively high jitter, some of the laser shots are lost. With a pulse energy of 1 mJ, a failure rate of up to 10% is observed.

Another method of switching the Pockels cells is to use an optically triggered avalanche transistor chain driving a Krytron pulser [5.13]. The rise time of the high-voltage pulse is on the order of 1 ns and the overall jitter of this electronic circuit has the same magnitude. Using a fast planar triode driver for the Pockels cells, the jitter of the high-voltage pulse can be reduced to less than 100 ps [5.14]. A jitter of the same order will also be obtained by using a Si or GaAs semiconductor switch which can be driven by microjoule pulses [5.15].

5.3.2 Beam Expansion

For expansion of the laser beam cross section along the beam path there are two methods available: the use of the natural beam divergence established by the cavity geometry of the oscillator or the use of optical recollimating systems.

The use of naturally diverging beams for increasing the beam diameter along a chain is suitable only for relatively small laser systems (up to output energies of approximately 100 J). Restricting this method to smaller systems is based upon the fact that in such systems the amplifiers are sufficiently short that the natural beam divergence of approximately one milliradian permits efficient use of the amplifiers' active volume (see Sect. 4.2.1). The maximum allowable intensity or beam loading is limited in this case more severely since Fresnel diffraction effects enhance the peak intensities at the amplifier exit windows, thereby subjecting them to increased risk of damage. Plane-wave Fresnel diffraction can lead to a four-fold increase in peak beam intensities, thereby exceeding the maximum desired beam loading (see Sect. 5.3.3).

The use of optical recollimating systems has the advantage that they reduce the beam divergence in inverse proportion to the expansion ratio, and hence minimize divergence-related losses in the amplifiers. With Galilean recollimating systems, Fresnel diffraction effects still persist and the beam loading limit noted above also cannot be exceeded. It is necessary to reduce the optical feedback into the amplifiers by using AR surfaces on the recollimation lenses.

A further improvement of the optical recollimation system can be made by image relaying a spatially smooth intensity distribution successively through the laser chain [5.16, 17]. Within the region lying close to each successive relay plane, Fresnel diffraction effects are reduced with a concomitant smoothing of the diffraction-related intensity fluctuations in the beam. Typically, planes near the output windows of the laser amplifiers are chosen as the relay planes since it is at these locations that the laser intensity is highest and the need for a spatially homogeneous beam the greatest. In the case of the iodine laser, the principal utility of employing an image-relaying system is to reduce the Fresnel diffraction fringes at critical planes in the chain. In addition, for subnanosecond pulses the image relaying system can be used as spatial filters to reduce self-focusing effects in the laser system.

5.3.3 Damage Thresholds of Optical Components

All the optical components in the laser chain require coatings or surface processing to either enlarge or reduce their reflectivities. These components include:

1) Optically polished bare surfaces for Brewster angle windows.
2) Lenses and windows with AR surfaces to eliminate parasitic oscillations and to reduce losses.
3) Mirrors used for pointing and centring the beam.
4) Dielectric coated polarizers for Pockels cells and Faraday rotators.

The most critical problem associated with these optical components is the occurence of laser induced damage. Damage threshold measurements have been carried out at λ = 1.064 µm but relatively few measurements have been made at λ = 1.315 µm. These damage measurements at λ = 1.315 µm have shown, however, that the damage thresholds at 1.064 µm and 1.315 µm are similar. The following summary of damage threshold values is derived from measurements made at λ = 1.064 µm and are believed to be generally applicable to λ = 1.315 µm as well.

1) *Optically-Polished Bare Surfaces.* Bare surfaces are primary used in iodine laser chains for Brewster angle windows. For 1-ns pulse duration and commercially polished bare surfaces, median damage thresholds $e_d \sim 16$ J/cm^2 were measured by LOWDERMILK and MILAM [5.2]. For pulse widths lying between 0.17 and 3.2 ns the pulse width dependence of the damage threshold varied approximately as $\sqrt{\tau_p}$. Caution should be employed when extrapolating these results beyond the measured pulse duration interval.

2) *Anti-Reflective Surfaces.* There are presently two principal types of anti-reflective surfaces: dielectric AR coatings and graded index surfaces.

Since for *dielectric AR coatings* the principle of operation is based upon destructive interference, the electric field intensities within the coatings are higher here than in other types of coatings, leading to correspondingly lower damage thresholds. If such dielectric AR coatings are used for amplifier windows, only protected hard coatings can be employed, otherwise a chemical reaction between the coating and the photolysis products of the laser medium will take place. According to the measurements reported in [5.2],the median damage threshold for four-layer silica/titania coatings with an undercoating of silica and "bowl-fed" polished substrate surfaces was for 1-ns pulses ~8J/cm^2. For conventionally polished substrate surfaces the damage threshold fell to ~5J/cm^2. The pulse width dependence appears to be nearly linear from 1 to 6 ns (varying in this range from 8 to 14 J/cm^2), then increasing more rapidly for pulse widths greater than 6 ns.

The *graded index surfaces* have proved to have significantly higher damage thresholds at λ = 1.06 µm than dielectric AR coatings. The graded index technique relies upon the gradual reduction of the substrate refractive index in the vicinity of the dielectric interface by increasing the porosity of the surface. There are presently three techniques being investigated for generating a suitable graded index surface.

a) Etching of special 2-phase glass. Median damage thresholds of $e_d \sim 12$ J/cm^2 have been measured with 1 ns pulses, but these surfaces exhibit excessive wave-front distortions produced by inhomogeneous etching as well as having a generally friable surface [5.18]. Considerable technical difficulties are also associated with the problem of producing high quality 2-phase glass disks of large aperture. The pulse width dependence of the damage threshold has not as yet been determined.

b) Etching of sol-gel layers. This process can be used on ordinary BK7 substrates, but the mechanical properties of the surfaces are not yet satisfactory. Although measurements have indicated median damage thresholds of $e_d \sim 21$ J/cm^2 [5.19] (for 1-ns pulses), the etched sol-gel technique has not been as yet extensively proven. Again the pulse width dependence has not been established.

c) Neutral solution processing [5.20]. This method appears to be the most promising because it achieves median damage thresholds of $e_d \sim 12$ J/cm^2 (for 1-ns pulse duration), uses ordinary substrates (such as BK-7), does not impair the optical quality of the treated components, and produces a surface with mechanical properties superior to both of the previous techniques. No pulse width dependence has yet been measured.

All of the graded index surfaces are by their very nature porous, and when used as windows on iodine laser amplifiers, they can absorb molecular iodine which may destroy the anti-reflection effect. This problem is perhaps not a serious one since the laser beam itself may serve to expel absorbed I_2 from the window surface. Furthermore, if the windows were to be maintained at a higher temperature than the remainder of the amplifiers, less I_2 would be absorbed. At the present time, no practical experience with graded index AR surfaces installed in iodine laser amplifiers has been obtained.

3) *High-Reflectivity (HR) Surfaces*. The large aperture pointing and centring mirrors must be high-reflectivity multilayer dielectric coated optics in order to withstand high beam loadings. Since the standing wave ratio of the electric field within the HR coatings is less than that in AR coatings,

their median damage threshold is found to be significantly higher and is not strongly influenced by the methods used to polish the substrates. This latter property follows obviously from the fact that the intensities reaching the substrate through the HR coating are much less than those incident on the substrates of AR-coated transmissive optics.

For a 15 layer stack of alternating silica/titania layers with a half-wave silica overcoat a median damage threshold $e_d \sim 15.0$ J/cm^2 was determined [5.2]. A similar dielectric stack without the silica overcoat showed a damage threshold $e_d \sim 8.5$ J/cm^2, all measurements here being made at 1-ns pulse duration and 1.06-μm wavelength. For pulses ranging in length from 0.17 to 3.2 ns, the damage threshold increased with the pulse length with the exponent lying between 0.5 and 1.0. The exponent was further found to vary from sample to sample. Extrapolation to pulse durations lying outside the 0.17- to 3.2-ns range cannot be made reliably.

For the case in which these laser mirrors would be used to supply diagnostic beams by transmitting small fractions of the incident laser light, it is necessary to use mirror substrates of sufficient internal quality so that the phase homogeneity of the transmitted beam is not impaired.

4) *Dielectric-Coated Polarizers*. These polarizers are used in concert with Pockels cells or Faraday rotators for the optical isolation between adjacent laser amplifiers and for protection of components from laser light retro-reflected from the target. The damage thresholds of dielectric-coated polarizers depend upon the polarization of the incident light. For "p"-polarized light the median damage threshold is $e_d \sim 4$ J/cm^2 (comparable to the AR-coated surfaces) whereas for the "S" polarization, the median damage threshold is $e_d \sim 8$ J/cm^2 (comparable to HR-coated surface) [5.21], all measurements being made with 1-ns pulse durations. The pulse dependence of the damage threshold has not yet been determined.

The foregoing discussion regarding survivability of optical coatings or graded index surfaces applies only when stringent measures have been taken by the manufacturer of the substrates and by the vendor applying the coatings to assure that the utmost cleanliness and purity of the materials have been used. In addition, it is recommended that coated or surface-processed optics be placed in irradiation enviroments not exceeding roughly half of their measured median damage thresholds. This safety factor is necessary because of unavoidable intensity fluctuations in the laser beam. In the preceding chapters the operating conditions specified for the iodine laser adhere to this conservative criterion.

5.3.4 Optical Isolation of Amplifiers and Prepulse Suppression

The requirement of optimal energy extraction from an amplifier chain calls for small-signal amplification exceeding the actual energy amplification by several orders of magnitude owing to the saturation of the laser medium. In the amplifier chain stringent measures have to be taken to suppress parasitic oscillations. Because of the high small-signal amplification, special precautions are also required to prevent prepulse signals, usually amplified at the full small-signal gain, from exceeding such a power level that sensitive targets are damaged before being struck by the main pulse.

There are several methods of effecting prepulse suppression and achieving high threshold values for external parasitic oscillations. As most of these methods satisfy both requirements simultaneously, both aspects will be discussed in parallel. However, before describing the measures for keeping the prepulse energy at a low level, its different sources have to be described first.

1) There is the background radiation from the oscillator, which passes through the pulse selection system during its opening time. This contribution depends on the oscillator behaviour. It still has not yet been measured with any iodine laser system in use, but experiments performed with the ASTERIX III laser indicate that this energy is less than 1 mJ on target, corresponding to a few nJ behind the oscillator.

2) The second contribution is due to the leaking of oscillator pulses through the closed pulse selection system. This leaking energy can be limited to a few μJ on target by using a pulse selection system with a high contrast ratio ($\geqq 10^9$) and by the use of saturable absorbers incorporated in the amplifier chain.

3) The prepulse energy caused by amplified spontaneous fluorescence radiation is of minor importance because of the small Einstein coefficient for spontaneous emission and the short pumping time of the amplifiers (up to 15 μs). It can be controlled by Pockels cells and by saturable absorbers.

4) The major portion of the prepulse energy results from parasitic oscillations in the amplifiers. It will be kept at a sufficiently low level (μJ on target) by satisfactory optical isolation of the amplifiers from each other and by operating the amplifiers at a small-signal amplification level which is about one order of magnitude below the threshold for internal parasitic oscillations.

The methods applied for amplifier decoupling and hence prepulse reduction are as follows:

1) The simplest procedure is to use large distances between adjacent amplifiers because parasitic oscillations result from diffuse reflection from windows and other external structures. Beam with divergences less than 1 mrad provide distances long enough for effective decoupling. This method is applicable only for small systems (<100 J). Larger laser chains may also utilize the advantage of small mutual solid angle subtense with the introduction of spatial filters and concomitant image relaying using suitable recollimating telescopes.

2) Further decoupling of the amplifiers will be obtained by placing stops at the entrance and exit aperture of each amplifier, with diameters chosen such that the zones covered by the shock waves are blocked. As these outer zones have the highest inversion densities, the stops reduce parasitic oscillations in the amplifiers and hence this contribution to the prepulse energy.

3) More effective amplifier decoupling and prepulse reduction will be obtained by placing a Pockels cell with polarizers between two adjacent amplifiers. As only KD*P Pockels cells with diameters of up to a few centimetre are currently available, these cells are mainly used for preamplifier isolation. For cells with diameters of several centimetre, contrast ratios of up to about 10^2 can be obtained, whereas for apertures in the millimetre range, specially selected Pockels cells can provide a contrast ratio of up to 10^5 when used with high-quality Glan-air prisms. They are most conveniently gated by the short (~1-ns) high-voltage pulse operating the pulse selection system. For exact timing, a delay line corresponding to the beam path length has to be used.

4) Saturable absorbers serve mainly for prepulse suppression; their isolation capability is correspondingly higher when their bandwidth exceeds that of the laser transition in the adjacent amplifiers. For the saturating transition at 1.3 μm, the lasing transition in absorption can be used [5.22, 23]. For this purpose the atomic iodine in the ground state can be produced by thermal dissociation of I_2 molecules in a hot quartz cell ($T \cong 800°C$). For nanosecond pulses the saturation characteristic is shown in Fig. 5.9 [5.10]. The ratio of the small-signal to saturated transmission is nearly 10^{-3}. As the saturation energy density is approximately 1 J/cm^2, the laser beam cross-section usually has to be compressed to insure saturated

transmission. Owing to the non-linear nature of the absorption, pulse shaping effects such as steepening and shortening of the pulse will take place [5.10]. Other non-linear effects, such as self-induced transparency or resonant self-focusing [5.24] were not observed since the condition of incoherent interaction $T_{2,abs} \leqq \tau_p$ was met.

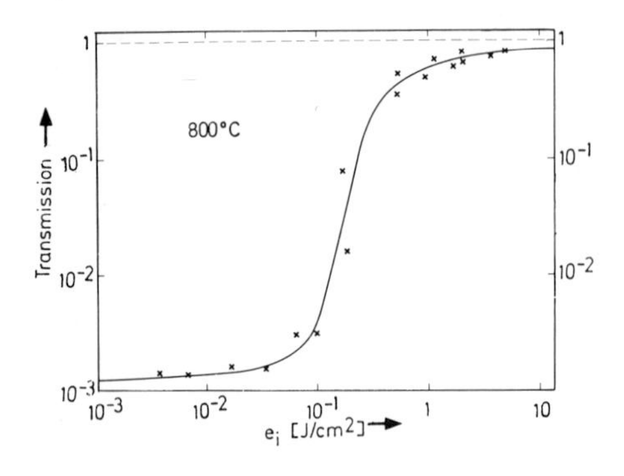

Fig. 5.9. Transmission of a saturable absorber cell (l = 40 cm, Ø 2,5 cm) filled with 50 mg I_2 at a temperature of 800°C [5.21]

The isolation capability is, however, restricted because the absorption bandwidth of this absorber (0.5-2.5 GHz [5.25]) is much smaller than the bandwidths of the amplifiers (5-20 GHz).

Special dyes such as BDN II [5.26,], Jul 2 [5.27] and a dye of unknown composition used in [5.28] have been investigated in different solutions for their ability for providing saturable absorber action at 1.3 μm. Regarding the qualification of BDN II as a saturable absorber, there are two opposing views [5.29,30]. From our experience Jul 2 dissolved in 1,2 dichloro-benzene turns out to be the best choice [5.31]. For this absorber the saturation intensity transmission T_{sa} is approximated for ~ 1-ns pulses by the empirical formula $T_{sa} = T_{ss}^{1/6}$, where T_{ss} is the small-signal intensity transmission. This formula yields a saturation transmission of 85% at a small-signal transmission of 20%. The explanation of this saturation behaviour requires the assumption of a three- or four-level energy scheme. As the ground-state repopulation time is in the subnanosecond region and the absorption cross-sections are about 10^{-16} cm^2, the saturation intensity is in the range of 0.1 GW/cm^2. The bandwidth of the saturation transition greatly exceeds the bandwidth of the amplifiers. Its isolation capability therefore corresponds to its prepulse suppression ability. This saturable dye has the advantage that less pulse shortening takes place than in an iodine absorber cell (see Fig. 3.12).

5) Faraday rotators also have amplifier decoupling capabilities. The optical isolation is proportional to the square root of the backward-forward extinction ratio. For present Faraday rotators this ratio can be as great as 10^3, depending on the homogeneity of the magnetic field and the quality of the polarizers. Their main function is, however, to protect sensitive laser components from being destroyed by laser light retro-reflected from the target. For this purpose the iodine laser, unlike other high-power lasers, only needs one Faraday rotator per arm, because there is only a small amplification of the retro-reflected light by the residual inversion stored in the amplifiers. This is due to the fact, that the retro-reflected light is spectrally broadened ($\Delta\lambda$ = 1 nm) and Doppler shifted, so that only a small fraction falls inside the amplification bandwidth of the laser medium ($\Delta\lambda$ = 0.15 nm).

5.4 Diagnostics for Iodine Lasers

Photodetector technology in the spectral region near 1.3 μm has only been developed to a modest level. This is evidenced by the fact that even recent reviews of infrared detectors [5.32] do not take the spectral region around 1.3 μm fully into account. Since, however, applications in the field of optical communications have aroused increasing interest in this region of the spectrum, an improvement in this situation can be expected [5.33, 34].

The following sections deal mainly with two topics:

- temporal resolution of pulses down to the region of about 100 ps, and
- spatial resolution of spatial intensity and transverse energy density distributions.

Since most of the calorimetric measurements tend to be independent of wavelength, no unique device for energy measurements is required for iodine laser energy measurements. Thus calorimeters used for the measurement of glass laser output energies can also be employed for the iodine laser.

5.4.1 Time-Resolved Diagnostics

Pulses with durations as short as 100 ps can be monitored either with a fast photodetector feeding into an oscilloscope (rise times as short as 90 ps can be displayed with the fastest equipment) or, more easily, by advanced technologies such as streak cameras. Both methods are described in this section.

Fast detectors can be based on two principal effects: internal photoeffect in semiconductors and external photoemission from special surfaces.

The internal photoeffect involves generation of charge carriers by photons, and their subsequent collection by means of an electric field in semiconductors. For selected geometries this effect is fast enough to be used for measuring light pulse lengths in the subnanosecond range. Photodetection schemes based on the photovoltaic effect normally provide the shortest response time for a given material. Appropriate techniques are avalanche, PIN, and Schottky barrier diodes. Suitable samples commercially available are made from Ge or GaAs, which exhibit spectral sensitivities peaking in the neighbourhood of 1.3 μm. Rise times down to 120 ps at sensitivities of up to 0.4 A/W have been reported [5.32]. Detectors exhibiting short response times must have a small sensitive area which, in turn, prohibits high pulse currents. As a consequence, reasonable signals are well below 100 mV into a 50-Ω termination. Signals at such a low voltage level cannot be displayed reliably on an ultrafast oscilloscope which usually combines a low sensitivity with a high bandwidth (>2 GHz). To facilitate interpretation of a signal produced by such a semiconductor device, the detector should respond linearly to the incident light intensity over at least one order of magnitude. This requirement, however, is satisfied only by selected samples. In spite of their moderate sensitivity of 0.03 V/MW, photon drag detectors made of GaAs or Si [5.35] may be of some interest for special applications since they afford a large sensitive area at a fairly short response time of about 1 ns in a coaxial arrangement.

Devices using the external photoelectric effect are based upon the absorption of the incident photons by the photocathode, the emission of electrons, and the subsequent acceleration of these electrons in an electric field. The most extensively used fast detector of this type is the vacuum photodiode equipped with an S-1 photocathode (diffused Ag-O-Cs layers) [5.36]. Its low sensitivity of 0.7 mA/W at 1.06 μm (max. 2.5 mA/W at 800 nm) drops further by a factor of nearly 300 to typically 2.5 μA/W at 1.3 μm (Fig. 5.10) [5.37, 38]. Additionally, this low sensitivity may vary from sample to sample within an order of magnitude as well as varying locally within the cathode area for a given sample by a factor of at least two [5.39]. However, this low and spatially inhomogeneous sensitivity is compensated by two advantages. Namely, by a rise time as low as 60 ps in specially designed arrangements [5.40] and signal amplitudes exceeding 10 V which facilitate reliable application of the detectors in an electrically

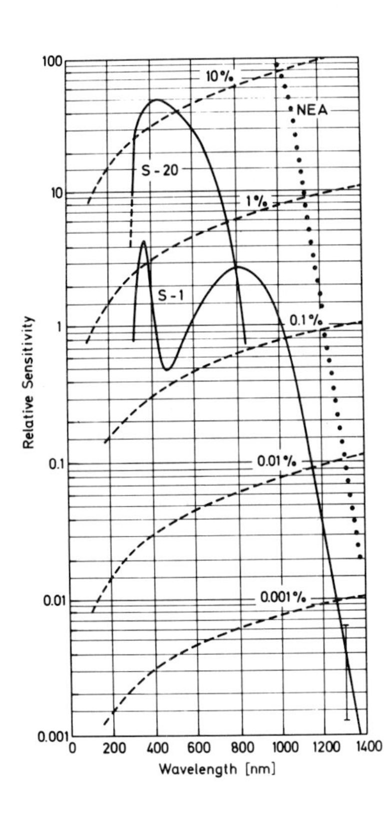

Fig. 5.10. Relative sensitivities of various photocathodes

noisy environment. At high output signals, care has to be taken to avoid radiation damage by hot spots. Selected samples show a linear response over several orders of magnitude, whereas usually the output signal follows the light intensity according to a power law with exponents ranging between 1 and 2.

Much higher sensitivity can be obtained by the photomultiplier principle which uses electron multiplication to increase the output signal. Pulses at power levels much less than a few watts can thus be detected and such devices are especially employed for prepulse detection. Special types of photomultipliers exhibit response times as short as 120 ps at amplification factors of up to 10^4 (static crossed field photomultiplier, Varian VM 148). In any application, however, it has to be determined if the technical advantages justify the high costs.

For a time resolution down to 10 ps, streak cameras equipped with an S-1 streaking tube have to be employed [5.41]. In the analysis of the displayed streaks, measurement of time intervals is usually more accurate than measurement of pulse shapes. This is due to the following reasons:

- nonlinear response of the cathode at the photon fluxes usually needed,
- small dynamic range of less than 1 : 5, and
- spatially varying sensitivity across the cathode [5.42, 43].

Although occasionally a marked decrease of the tube qualities during storage is observed, there are selected tubes which exhibit nearly unaltered performance for several years. Improvements so far suffer from a lack of detailed knowledge about the actual physical processes involved in the release of electrons by photons in the complex Ag-O-Cs layers. At the moment, however, the production of modern compact streak tubes with S-1 cathodes has been ceased world wide. For the future it may be expected that the S-1 photocathode with its low sensitivity at 1.3 μm will be replaced by NEA cathodes made from negative electron affinity materials such as GaAsInP [5.44], which shows a sensitivity roughly 50 times higher than the S-1 photocathode at 1.3 μm (Fig. 5.10). A change in this unfortunate situation may occur with the development of the so-called crystal streak camera [5.45]. The working principle of such a streak camera is based on electro-optical deflection of the beam during its passage through an appropriate non-linear crystal such as KDP. Recent data suggests a spectral response range from 0.4 to 4 μm and a time resolution of 40 ps.

Besides using the internal (semiconductor devices) and external (photomultipliers and similar devices) photoeffects for detecting iodine laser radiation, detectors based upon heat sensing have also been utilized for measuring short laser pulses. Tiny pyroelectric detectors allow the measurement of pulses with rise times less than 1 ns, but at the expense of the responsivity, which is then of the order of 10^{-5} V/W.

The low sensitivity of S-1 photocathodes at 1.3 μm can be overcome by second harmonic generation (SHG) of the iodine laser radiation. Use can then be made of vacuum photodiodes and related devices employing the high-performance S-20 photocathode which exhibits a fairly high sensitivity of 70 mA/W at the SHG wavelength of 657 nm. Compared with detection at the fundamental wavelength, this method can yield a sensitivity enhanced by a few orders of magnitude even at a SHG conversion efficiency of less than 1%. Linearity, dynamic range and spatially homogeneous sensitivity favour S-20 cathodes. A disadvantage of the procedure arises from the fact that fairly well collimated light has to be used for SHG. Otherwise the overall SHG conversion efficiency drastically decreases. However, for pulses emitted by a typical iodine oscillator this condition is not critical. The method has been successfully applied using $LiIO_3$. There was no evidence of pulse shape deformation in the SHG process.

5.4.2 Spatially Resolved Diagnostics

For a number of experimental investigations with iodine lasers, knowledge of the spatial intensity distribution across the beam is required. Examples are corrections of wave-front distortions to avoid deterioration of the focusibility and measurements of intensity dependent parameters with an extended beam.

The purpose of this section is to summarize briefly the techniques that have been successfully employed in iodine laser diagnostics. Common to all methods is the feature that the recorded distributions are integrated over the pulse length. For rapid, qualitative analysis, burn patterns supply approximate information. Possible beam recording materials are unexposed and developed polaroids, exposed and developed X-ray films, and UV recording paper. With some experience it is even possible to obtain an order of magnitude estimate of the intensity using these burn patterns. To afford transient visualization of iodine laser beam patterns, the Kodak IR phosphor chart may be used [5.46].

For quantitative determination of transverse distributions, more complicated techniques, such as detector arrays, IR television and IR photography, have to be used. Arrays of Ge detectors or pyrodetectors can be applied to measure energy density distributions. Their main advantages are a high degree of linearity and a large dynamic range.

If a two-dimensional display of the transverse distribution is required, TV systems represent a valuable tool. Peripheral equipment such as recording or information processing electronics considerably broadens the field of their applications. Vidicons with a PbS/PbO target, which have a reasonable sensitivity between 350 and 1800 nm, or pyricons [5.47] covering the even broader range from the near to the far infrared are well developed.

A second possibility of two-dimensional recording of beam patterns is the use of photographic material. For applications which require only a limited dynamic range, Kodak high-speed infrared film or infrared colour film can be applied. Much better results have been achieved by hypersensitized Kodak I-Z plates [5.48]. The hypersensitization procedure [5.49] increases the infrared sensitivity by a factor of up to 460. Measurements of the optical density as a function of intensity revealed a linear dynamic range of 1 : 5. If the non-linear portions of the sensitivity curves are included, the dynamic range is extended to 1 : 10. In all applications of I-Z plates the energy density has to be kept below 0.5 J/cm^2 to avoid overexposure.

5.5 Frequency Conversion

Recent experiments have established that significant improvements in inverse Bremsstrahlung absorption and a reduction of fast electron preheat can be obtained if the target is irradiated with visible and near ultraviolet (UV) instead of infrared laser light [5.50-53]. Nearly all the major laser fusion facilities in the world are therefore finding it useful to modify their equipment to permit target irradiation experiments to be conducted at wavelengths shorter than 700 nm.

By generating higher harmonics of the fundamental iodine laser radiation at 1315 nm, high power pulses at wavelengths in the visible and near ultraviolet region of the spectrum can be obtained. Generation of second (SHG), third (THG), fourth (FHG), and higher harmonics can be achieved with high conversion efficiencies (up to 80%) in non-linear crystals.

SHG of iodine laser pulses in KDP, KD*P, and $LiIO_3$ was first applied to the measurement of pulse durations [5.54,55]. Later, efficient generation of second, third, and fourth harmonics was demonstrated [5.56]. KD*P turned out to be the most useful non-linear material for SHG work with iodine lasers because of its low absorption at 1.3 μm, high damage threshold, and availability in large sizes.

An advantage possessed by the iodine laser from the standpoint of target irradiation experiments is that the fourth harmonic falls at a wavelength of 329 nm. This wavelength is shorter than the third harmonic of the Nd-glass laser and yet still permits the use of moderate priced fused silica optics. The present status of iodine laser conversion experiments as well as some relevant parameters are given in Table 5.1. These are preliminary results only based upon the initial experiments. In principle, performances and conversion efficiencies similar to those obtained already with Nd-glass lasers [5.57] can be expected for the iodine laser as well since the non-linear coefficients and damage thresholds of KD*P and KDP for the corresponding wavelengths are very nearly the same. The relatively low FHG conversion efficiency listed in Table 5.1 is due to relatively poor beam quality and a KDP quadrupling crystal with inadequate surface finish and relatively high scattering.

The conversion efficiencies quoted in the table were achieved at intensities ranging from 1.5 to 3 GW/cm^2. Maximum conversion into the third harmonic was achieved with the "polarization mismatch" scheme described by CRAXTON [5.58].

For FHG, a commercial KDP doubler crystal originally designed for use with a 694-nm ruby laser was used, since the second harmonic of the iodine laser (658 nm) lies in the vicinity of the ruby laser wavelength.

It should be noted that the phase-matching angles in KD*P depend on the amount of deuteration. With decreasing deuteration, the phase-matching angle increases monotonically towards the phase-matching angle for KDP. Thus, for 0% deuteration, the phase matching angle is 62°, whereas for 100% deuteration, the angle decreases to 52°. The amount of deuteration necessary in a KD*P crystal depends on the particular application. According to [5.59], the absorption at 1315 nm is 2.5%/cm for 98.9% deuteration and 6%/cm for 87% deuteration. (The corresponding value for KDP is 30%/cm.) Under the assumption that in the region of high deuteration the damage threshold does not vary significantly with deuteration, it is apparent that 90% deuteration is adequate in single-shot operation. When a high repetition rate is required, however, the deuteration should be as high as possible to avoid runaway of the phase-matching angle by a temperature rise in the crystal.

The experiments summarized in Table 5.1 were performed with beams having diameters ranging from 5 to 8 mm. Extension to beams of larger diameter is straightforward. For example, 60% conversion for SHG was demonstrated with a beam 4 cm in diameter.

Table 5.1. Present status and relevant parameter for iodine laser radiation conversion experiments. The phase matching angles listed for KD*P are for 99% deuteration

	Units	SHG	THG	FHG
Generated Wavelength	[nm]	657.6	438.4	328.8
Crystal		KD*P	KD*P	KDP
Phase-Matching Angle	[deg]	51.5	46.0	53.6
Crystal Type		II	II/II	I/II
Conversion Efficiency	[%]	70	50	15

For target irradiation experiments conducted with second harmonic light at 658 nm, efficient supression of the fundamental wavelength at 1315 nm is required. Since the use of a prism is awkward at large beam diameters, and beam separation using polarizers is not feasible for Type-II harmonic conversion crystals, filters or narrow-band dielectric HR mirrors have to be used to eliminate the 1315-nm radiation from the beam incident on the target chamber. In the case of the iodine laser, infrared absorbing filters are available which transmit approximately 80% at 658 nm, while attenuating the fundamental beam at 1315 nm by a factor of 100. Superior rejections of the fundamental can be obtained with dichroic mirrors. With the present state of the art, 99.5% reflectivity can be achieved at 657 nm while keeping the reflectivity at 1315 nm down to only 5%. An arrangement of four such mirrors reduces the fundamental by more than a factor of 10^5 while delivering some 98% of the incident second harmonic radiation at 658 nm to the target chamber.

6. The ASTERIX III System

The realization of a high power iodine laser will now be illustrated by describing the layout of the single-beam ASTERIX III laser, built at the Max-Planck-Institut für Quantenoptik, Garching [6.1-4]. This laser has been in routine use for laser plasma research since 1978 and has already demonstrated that it meets the requirements of high-quality target experiments. The ASTERIX III laser is presently capable of delivering an output power higher than 1 TW at an energy level of up to 300 J and pulse lengths ranging from 180 to 360 ps. Its present overall efficiency (defined as the laser output energy over the electrical energy stored in the capacitor banks) is 0.08%.

6.1 Technical Features

A schematic of ASTERIX III is shown in Fig. 6.1. The main components of this system are the oscillator, the pulse selection system and four amplifiers. A saturable absorber serves for prepulse suppression and a Faraday rotator protects sensitive laser components from being destroyed by light retro-reflected from the target.

Several components serve for beam diagnostics, laser control and remote alignment of the laser beam. The laser is situated in a temperature- ($\pm$ 1°C) and humidity-controlled room.

6.1.1 Oscillator and Pulse Selection System

The oscillator operating in the TEM_{00} mode in a semiconfocal resonator is acousto-optically mode-locked. Its cavity length of 258.2 cm corresponds to the modulator frequency of 27.1 MHz (Sect. 3.1.2). It is mounted on a granite bench. To achieve subnanosecond pulses reliably, the fused silica modulator is powered in pulsed operation by a 20-W RF pulse (pulse

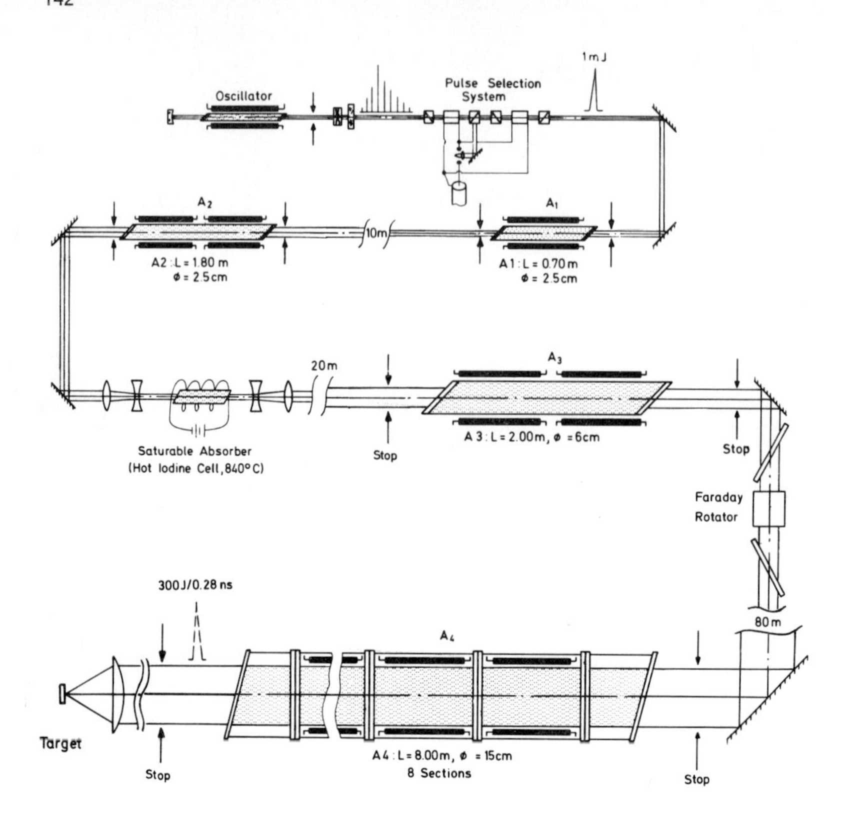

Fig. 6.1. Schematic of the ASTERIX III laser

length 1 ms), thus providing a modulation index of about 1 [6.5]. The reflectivity of the output mirror is 60%. Further information regarding the dimensions of the laser tube, the pressure of the laser medium and the specifications of the pumping system are given in Table 6.1.

The oscillator emits a train of pulses with lengths in the range of 0.75 ns (FWHM) which are exclusively on the 3-4 transition. The single pulse separated by the pulse selection system has an energy in the range of 1 mJ and a diffraction-limited beam divergence of 8×10^{-4} rad (full angle).

The pulse selection system provides high optical isolation of the oscillator from the amplifier chain. It consists of two Pockels cells in series and three Glan polarizers, the total attenuation of the closed system (zero voltage at the Pockels cells) being about 10^{-9}. The Pockels cells are switched by a laser-triggered spark gap.

Table 6.1. Specifications of the oscillator and the amplifiers

	Units	Osc.	A_1	A_2	A_3	A_4
Active length	[cm]	85	65	160	185	740
Active diameter	cm	0.8	1.6	1.6	5.5	15.5
Number of pumping sections		2	1	2	2	8
C_3F_7I pressure	mbar	155	80	80	33	12
Argon pressure	bar	0.92	0.65	1.3	2.6	3.2
Total number of flashlamps		4	4	4	16	64
Active length of the flashlamps	cm	43	65	79	92	92
Inner diameter of the flashlamps	cm	0.8	0.8	0.8	1.8	1.8
Xe pressure	mbar	40	40	40	40	40
Max. operating voltage	kV	45	40	40	40	40
Electr. energy stored per amplifier at max. pumped energy	kJ	1.1	2.6	4.4	76	306
Number of circuits		1	1	1	8	32
Input energy/flashlamp	kJ	0.28	0.66	1.1	4.8	4.8
Current pulse width (FWHM)	μs	1.1	2.4	2.4	5.5	5.5
Rise time of the pumping light	μs	1.0	1.6	1.6	4.2	4.2
Pumping time until extraction	μs	1.5	6.0	6.0	11.5	11.5
Trigger delay	μs	10.0	5.5	5.5	0	0
Max. stored inversion energy at pulse passage	[J]	1	2.6	7.3	90	890

6.1.2 Amplifiers

The pulse to be amplified passes four amplifiers of successively increasing diameter, length and stored inversion energy. The distance between the individual amplifiers is chosen such that the beam which has a divergence of about 1 mrad fits the diameter of the following amplifiers. The beam expansion is established up to the saturable absorber by the natural divergence of the oscillator and then by the telescope placed between the saturable absorber and the third amplifier. The beam diameter thereby increases from 0.2 to 15 cm over a distance of 150 m.

The first and second amplifiers serve as preamplifiers. They are assembled from one quartz tube and pumped by four flashlamps operated in parallel. The main amplifiers are arranged from two and eight sections, respectively, each section having eight flashlamps powered by one capacitor bank. The dimensions of the amplifier quartz tubes, the number and dimensions of the flashlamps and the specifications of the capacitor banks are given in Table 6.1.

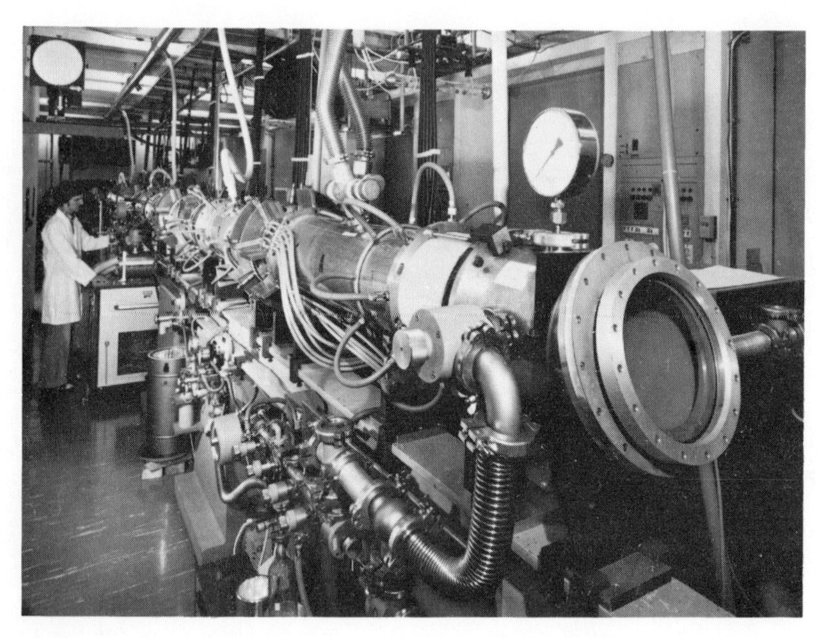

Fig. 6.2. Fourth amplifier of the ASTERIX III laser

The largest energy gain of the pulse takes place in the fourth amplifier (Fig. 6.2). The inversion density profile of this amplifier, derived from measurements of the small-signal amplification, is shown in Fig. 6.3 at i-C_3F_7I partial pressures of 8 and 15 mbar. For laser operation an intermediate partial pressure of 12 mbar provides an appropriate gain profile. The inversion profiles of the other amplifiers correspond to that of the fourth amplifier. The inversion energy stored in the different amplifiers at maximum pumping energy available for pulse amplification is listed in

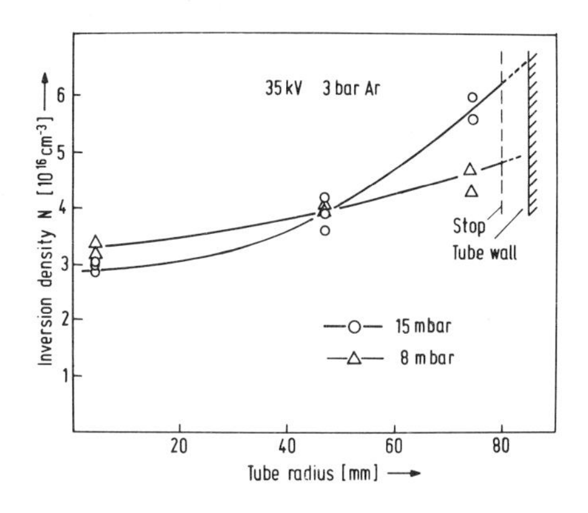

Fig. 6.3. Inversion density profile of the fourth amplifier at a i-C_3F_7I pressure of 8 mbar and 15 mbar after 12 μs pumping time

Table 6.1. For the windows of the amplifiers, BK-7 plates 1 to 3.5 cm thick are used. The reflectors of the preamplifiers and the main amplifiers are U shaped.

The regeneration systems for the laser media of the preamplifiers are built from aluminium storage vessels and glass or aluminium connecting pipes. The amplifiers with their regeneration systems can be evacuated to a pressure of 10^{-3} mbar. The amplifiers are cooled by an open-cycle air flow or by a closed loop He system. Stable temperature conditions can be established within 5 to 10 min., depending on the size of the amplifiers.

6.1.3 Components for Optical Isolation and Prepulse Suppression

The simultaneous requirements of high threshold values for the occurrence of external parasitic oscillations and low prepulse energies are met by different measures. First the large distances between the amplifiers provide a certain decoupling effect. This is enhanced by the stops placed at the entrance and the exit of each amplifier. These stops block the zones with the highest inversion density close to the amplifier wall which are affected by the shock waves.

Very effective oscillator-amplifier decoupling and prepulse suppression is achieved by the pulse selection system. Also the Faraday rotator placed between the third and fourth amplifiers serves for amplifier decoupling. Its backward-forward extinction ratio is 100.

Furthermore, the saturable iodine absorber installed with its beam compression and expanding elements between the second and third amplifiers, diminishes the small-signal amplification of the laser system by a factor of 10^3. It correspondingly reduces the contributions to the prepulse energy arising from the leaking of oscillator pulses through the closed pulse selection system and from the spontaneous emission of the first and second amplifiers. In order to maintain a sufficiently low saturation energy density, the absorption bandwidth of the absorber has to be much smaller than the gain bandwidth of the amplifiers (Sect. 5.3.3). Therefore its amplifier decoupling capability is restricted.

All these measures for optical amplifier decoupling and prepulse reduction provide the conditions in the ASTERIX III system that an overall small-signal amplification of all amplifiers of about 10^7 can be sustained with a sufficiently low prepulse energy (< 1 mJ) at an overall energy amplification of 5×10^5.

6.2 Laser Maintenance and Reliability of Operation

The maintenance effort for the ASTERIX III system in long-term operation is essentially restricted to replenishment of the laser medium in the storage vessels of the regeneration systems and replacement of flashlamps. With storage vessels of the present size the laser medium for the oscillator and the preamplifiers has to be refilled after 1500 to 2000 shots, and for the main amplifiers after 200 to 300 shots. Before replenishing, the condensed iodine has to be taken out. When the laser system is always operated at full load, the flashlamps of the oscillator and the preamplifiers have to be replaced after 1500 to 2000 shots, and those of the main amplifiers after about 1000 shots.

In daily operation the alignment of the system has to be checked before starting laser operation. This alignment procedure uses He-Ne beams coinciding with the iodine laser beam. As shown in Fig. 6.4, three He-Ne lasers are used for this purpose. To check the state of alignment, fiducial marks are placed in the beam paths. In addition, since the beam has to be folded several times, the He-Ne laser beam transmitted through the dielectric coatings of the mirrors is monitored behind these mirrors by an array of photodiodes. If necessary, the laser beam is then easily adjusted by remote mirror control.

The laser can be fired with a repetition rate of up to one shot every 10 min. In each shot the laser operation is checked by measuring the timing of the pumping processes and by recording the output energies after each amplifier. Furthermore, information on the pulse shape is provided

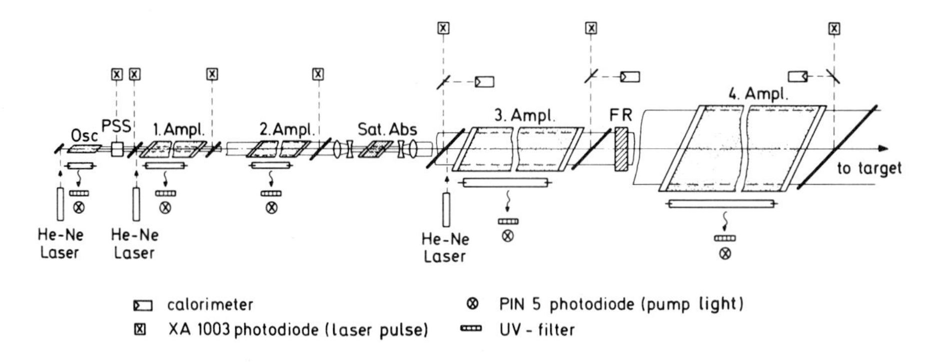

Fig. 6.4. Diagnostic system of the ASTERIX III laser

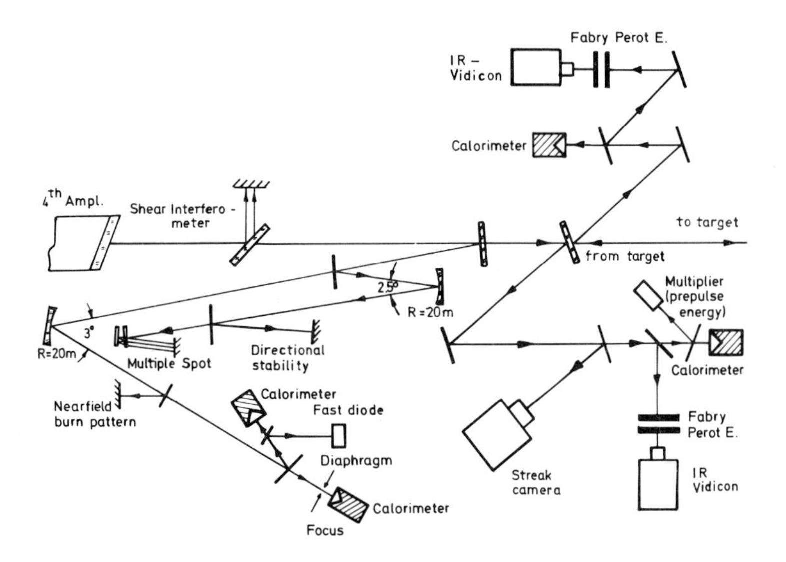

Fig. 6.5. Schematic setup of the diagnostics for the output pulse

at the output of the first amplifier by a fast diode, and at the output of the fourth amplifier by a streak camera with a S1 cathode (Figs. 6.4,5). In operating the laser it was established that the misfiring rate due to failure of the electrical system is 1% to 2%. Such cases of misfiring also include shots with a jitter exceeding 0.5 μs in the timing of the pumping process of the amplifiers. The highest fluctuations were measured in the pulse length. The fraction of the shots consisting of double pulses or pulses which differ in length from the average values by more than 50% is less than 6%. The fluctuations of the laser output energy were up to 5%.

6.3 Laser Performance

The diagnostics for the investigation of the output pulse properties of the ASTERIX III laser are shown in Fig. 6.5. Of primary interest are the energy and shape of the laser pulse, its prepulse energy and power, the beam quality (focusibility), the pulse bandwidth (temporal smoothness), the directional stability of the beam and its energy density profile.

6.3.1 Output Energy and Pulse Length

The maximum pulse energy obtained with a charging voltage of 40 kV for all amplifiers is 285 ± 15 J. As the entire system is pumped with an energy input of 370 kJ, the maximum pulse energy corresponds to an overall laser efficiency of η_o = 0.08%.

The mean pulse duration measured with the streak camera at the output of the fourth amplifier is 280 ps (FWHM). An output power of more than 1 TW can thus be achieved. During the amplification process the pulse shape is significantly modified. Substantial pulse steepening and shortening occurs in the saturable absorber, and to a lesser degree in the saturation region of the third and fourth amplifiers. As shown in Fig. 6.6, the pulse length decreases from 0.75 ns at the exit of the second amplifier to 0.28 ns (FWHM) after the fourth amplifier. Information on the reproducibility of the output pulse lengths are specified in the histogram Fig. 6.7, which is based on

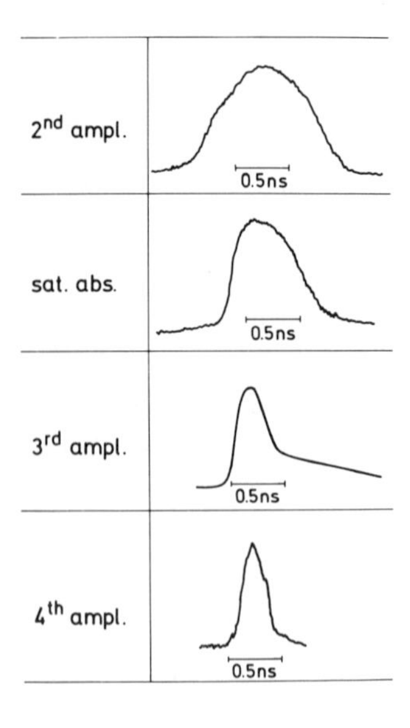

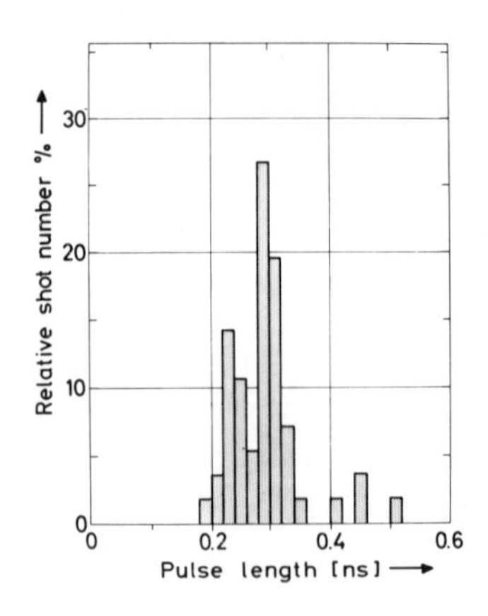

Fig. 6.7. Histogram of the pulse length

◁ Fig. 6.6. Time evolution of the pulse along the chain (streak camera measurements) streak camera measurements. The fluctuations in the output pulse lengths are mainly caused by fluctuations in the oscillator pulse.

The few pulses between 400 and 500 ps with a larger deviation from the average pulse length result from oscillator double pulses. Pulse statistics revealed that there is no significant correlation between output pulse length and energy in the energy range investigated (60 to 210 J).

According to theoretical investigations [6.6] in the range from 150 ps to a few ns the output energy should be independent from the pulse lengths. For pulses exceeding 10 ns an increase of the output energy due to hyperfine relaxation processes of the upper sublevels can be expected. For pulses below 150 ps, the output energy has to be reduced because of the damage threshold limitations of coatings.

6.3.2 Prepulse Power

The prepulse power is measured with a photomultiplier at a power contrast ratio of 3×10^{-10} and a rise time of 3.5 ns. The power detection threshold is 100 W and hence, due to the pumping time of 10 μs, only energies exceeding 1 mJ can be detected.

There are several contributions for the prepulse power on target (Sect. 5.3.3). The prepulse power contribution produced by the background radiation from the oscillator which may pass through the pulse selection system during its opening time (16 ns) has not yet been accurately measured because of the limitations in the time resolution of the detection system. But the target experiments performed with the ASTERIX III system give indirect experimental evidence that this energy is insufficient to affect the target. The contribution caused by the leaking of the oscillator pulses through the closed pulse selection system has been measured to be on the order of 1 kW. Because of the subnanosecond pulse lengths it will, however, only increase the prepulse energy by 2 μJ.

The measurement of the prepulse power showed that except for the oscillator prepulse leakage, all contributions, including the amplified spontaneous emission and the prelasing of the amplifiers, are below the power detection threshold (100 W). Owing to this threshold and the flashlamp pumping time of around 10 μs the total prepulse energy is less than 1 mJ. Even with a highly reflecting plane metal target carefully aligned with the focus of the target lens at normal incidence, no increase of the prepulse power could be detected.

6.3.3 Beam Quality

There are several sources which may lead to wave-front distortions of the laser beam. As described in Chap. 4, two groups can be distinguished. The first one covers the intensity-dependent sources; these are self-focusing due to n_2 (Sect. 4.1.1) and self-focusing or defocusing caused by spatially inhomogeneous gain saturation (Sect. 4.1.2). The second group comprises the intensity independent wave-front distortions; such sources are imperfect optical components, air turbulence along the beam path and spatially inhomogeneous pumping.

First the beam quality of the pulse was determined along the laser beam path by measuring the focusibility of the laser beam, and then the sources of the wave-front distortions were investigated. To evaluate the beam quality the multiple-spot and diaphragm methods were used (Fig. 6.5). In Fig. 6.8 the multiple-spot method is illustrated with an intensity profile recorded at the exit of the third amplifier. The results of the multiple-spot and diaphragm methods agree within the measuring accuracy. In Fig. 6.9 the ratio of the measured focal spot size to the ideal spot size is plotted versus the beam path length. The ideal reference spot size behind the os-

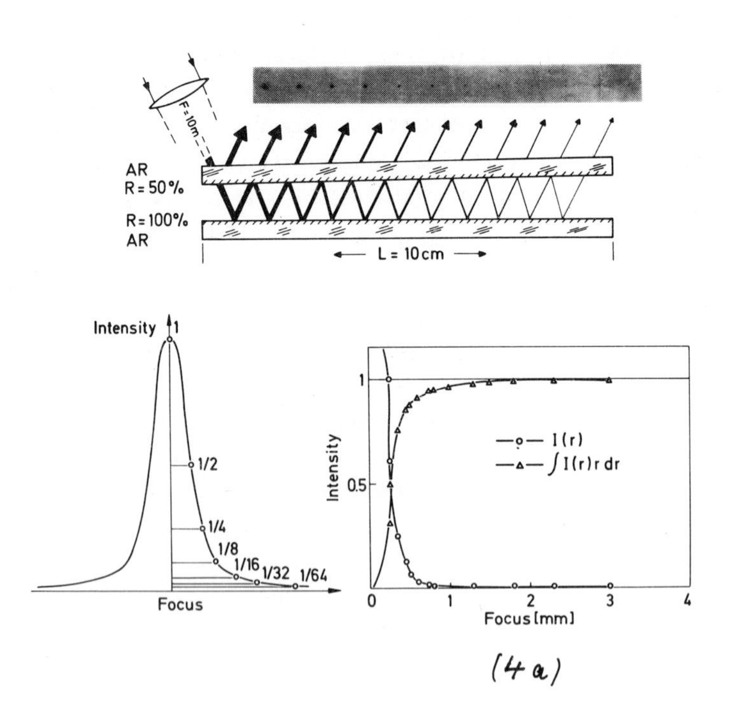

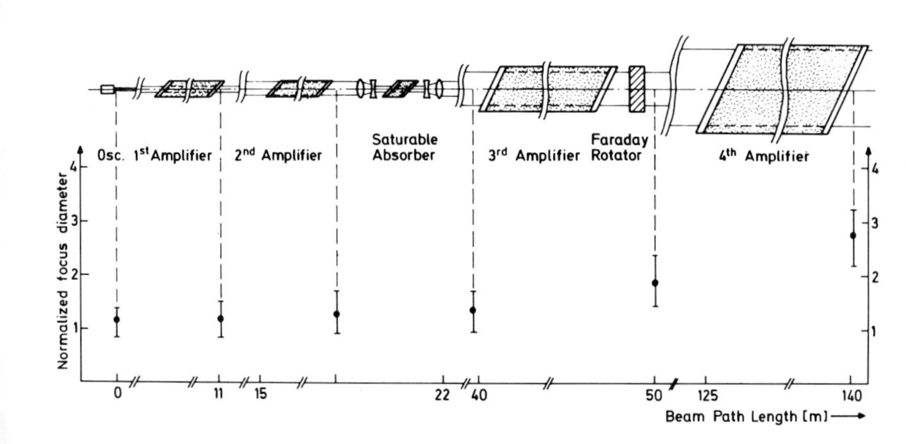

Fig. 6.9. Relative focal spot size at various locations along the laser chain

cillator and the first amplifier is the spot size of a Gaussian beam, and behind the other amplifiers an Airy spot size because of the increasingly rectangular spatial intensity profile of the beam. The experimental focal spot size was defined by the diameter containing 87% of the total energy. Its value has been measured at the exit of the fourth amplifier to be 2 to 3 times the ideal one. This means that an ideal f/2 lens can focus the beam to a spot size of 20 μm.

To determine the sources of the beam quality reduction, the focal spot size after the fourth amplifier was measured in the power range from 0.2 to 0.7 TW. No power dependence was detected. Thus the beam quality degradation is exclusively caused by intensity independent influences, such as imperfect optical components or optical inhomogeneities in the laser medium or in the air of the beam path.

To investigate these effects, lateral shearing interferograms were taken at different locations along the laser system. In Fig. 6.10 such an interferogram recorded in the horizontal direction of shear at the exit of the third amplifier is displayed. The wave-front distortion here is less than one wavelength. In the vertical direction it is of the same order of magnitude. Figure 6.11 shows an interferogram taken in the horizontal shear direction at the exit of the fourth amplifier. Here the maximum wave-front distortion does not exceed one wavelength. The interferograms vary from shot to shot indicating that the wave-front disturbances have a random nature. The disturbances therefore originate from optical inhomogeneities present in the laser medium or in the air beam path. A comparison of re-

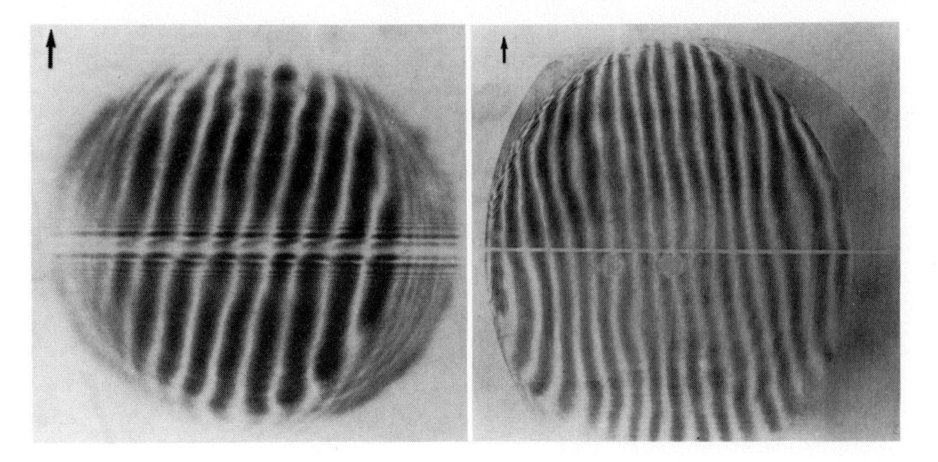

Fig. 6.10. Lateral shearing interferogram after the third amplifier

Fig. 6.11. Lateral shearing interferogram after the fourth amplifier

sults with and without the fourth amplifier in operation demonstrates that even the operation of the longest amplifier does not introduce additional wave front distortions. The beam quality reduction is therefore primarily caused by gasdynamic disturbances in the air between the amplifiers.

6.3.4 Energy Density Profile

The beam quality achieved in the ASTERIX III system implies a symmetric beam profile whose structure should be basically determined by diffraction. This expectation is confirmed by the near-field beam photograph taken at a distance of 10 m from the exit of the fourth amplifier (Fig. 6.12). The picture shows a symmetric structure with Fresnel rings but without any noticeable hot spots. The Fresnel rings originate from the hard stops placed at the entrances of the amplifiers.

A profile similar to the near-field diffraction pattern is also recorded by hypersensitized Kodak IZ plates in a plane equivalent to a position 400 μm in front of the focus of the f/2 target lens. Figure 6.13 shows the photometer curve of the profile. According to the inversion profile of the amplifiers, the energy density distribution has a convex Fresnel profile. Measurements of the intensity profile in the focus position displayed a soft and symmetric structure.

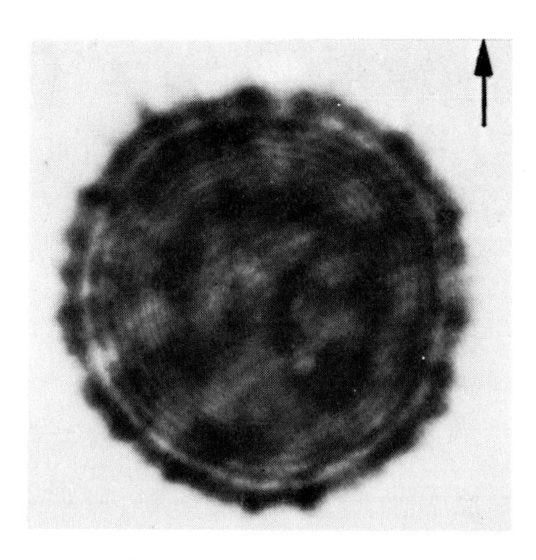

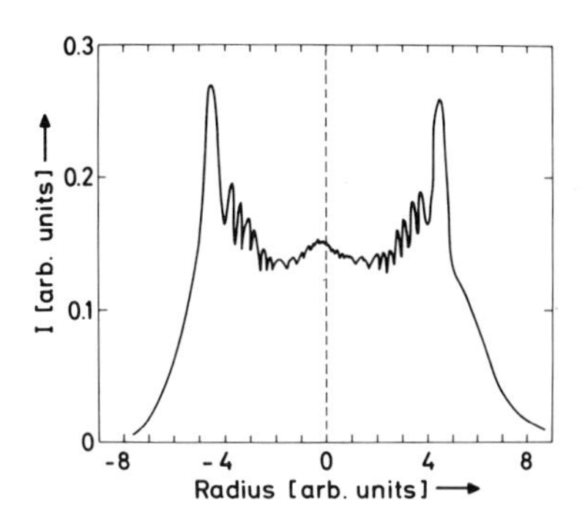

Fig. 6.13. Photometer curve of the energy density profile in a plane 400 μm ahead of the focus of the f/2 target lens

Fig. 6.12. Burn pattern of the beam taken 10 m behind the exit of the fourth amplifier

6.3.5 Pulse Bandwidth

It was necessary to further investigate whether the requirements of the target experiments regarding the temporal pulse smoothness are met by the iodine laser. For this purpose bandwidth measurements were performed with a Fabry-Perot interferometer. The subnanosecond pulse was investigated using spacers between the interferometer plates in the range from 1 to 12.5 cm. The interferogram is recorded by an infrared vidicon. Its evaluation yielded a pulse bandwidth of about $\Delta\nu$ = 2 GHz at a pulse length of τ = 280 ps. The bandwidth product $\Delta\nu\tau = 0.6$ implies that the pulse has no substructure. This is additionally supported by pulse shape measurements with an EPL ICC 512 streak camera at a time resolution of 20 ps/mm. The streak photographs showed a temporally smooth pulse without any substructure.

6.3.6 Spatial Focus Stability

The shot-to-shot stability of the laser focus position is of importance for pellet experiments. Scatter in the focus position in the axial beam direction can be caused in the amplifiers by a non-constant whole-beam lensing effect originating from inhomogeneous pumping or spatially non-uniform saturation. Measurements performed with an f/2 lens showed that the axial focus position remains within the measuring accuracy of $\pm$40 μm at the same position, irrespective of whether all the amplifiers were fired or only individual ones.

Focus position fluctuations transverse to the beam direction can originate from imperfect mechanical stability of mirrors and lenses and by varying temperature gradients transverse to the amplifier axis (Sect. 4.3.1). These gradients lead to a stronger beam deflection in the vertical direction than in the horizontal direction. The deviation in the vertical direction correlates quantitatively with the calculated deviations based on measured temperature gradients in the laser medium. This effect has been noticeably reduced by gas cooling the amplifier walls. Under such conditions the directional deviations of the laser beam in a series of shots are 20 μrad horizontally and 30 μrad vertically. This corresponds to a displacement of the focal spot centre in the horizontal direction of $\pm 10\%$ and in the vertical direction of $\pm 15\%$ of the focal spot size.

6.4 Potential for Improvements

The target experiments performed with the present design of the ASTERIX III system have proved the feasibility of the iodine laser for plasma experiments [6.7,8]. Regarding the focusibility of the laser beam, the prepulse power, the repetition rate, and the reliability of the laser system, these exacting requirements have been met. This fact does not imply that the laser has already reached its final state of development. There is still potential for further improvement of the following properties: beam focusibility, smoothness of the beam profile, pulse width flexibility, layout of the beam path, and extraction efficiency of the stored inversion energy.

Although an excellent beam focusibility has already been obtained, its quality can be further improved by diminishing the wave-front distortions caused by the optical inhomogeneities in the long air beam path between the amplifiers. These distortions can be substantially reduced by shielding the beam path. This can be done with least effort by shortening the space between adjacent amplifiers by means of optical beam expansion. Here the method of image relaying, as described in [6.9], offers the best prospects. By this method not only will the beam path length be shortened and partially shielded, but also the diffraction effects (Fresnel rings) caused by the hard stops placed at the entrances and exits of the amplifiers can be greatly reduced by appropriate imaging. Smooth beam profiles without strong variations in the loading can thus be obtained. Furthermore, if spatial filtering is employed between all amplifier stages (Sect. 5.4.2), coupling of adjacent amplifiers can be reduced and the value of the small--scale B integral can be controlled, allowing pulses with lengths of down to 150 ps to be amplified at the highest available energy level providing that sufficiently large f numbers for the spatial filters are selected.

With the ASTERIX III laser, an output pulse length in the range of only 0.15 to 0.5 ns can be generated. For future laser plasma experiments, however, pulses with lengths of up to a few nanoseconds should be made available. Since strong pulse compression occurs in the saturated amplifiers and absorbers of an iodine laser amplifier chain, the input pulse has to be smooth with a length of several nanoseconds. This requirement cannot be satisfied by the technique of mode locking. It can, however, be met when an excimer-laser-pumped iodine oscillator is applied [6.10].

A further increase of the output pulse pulse length can be obtained, when a Jul II saturable absorber is employed instead of an iodine absorber (Sect. 5.3.4). The use of a dye absorber has the additional advantage that it improves the optical isolation between adjacent amplifiers due to its broader absorption bandwidth and, moreover, it simplifies the beam path since the low saturation energy density of the dye does not require the installation of any beam compression elements. Disadvantageous are, however, the lower prepulse suppression ratio and the lower saturation transmission of the Jul II absorber. In order to obtain the same prepulse suppression ratio at the same energy level in the amplifier chain, the number of Jul II absorbers and the output energies of the preceeding amplifiers therefore have to be increased correspondingly.

There is furthermore potential for raising the laser efficiency. This can be achieved by an enhancement of the extraction efficiency of the optical energy stored in the amplifiers. In the present first design, the pulse to be amplified passes through the amplifier without saturating it. This fact is demonstrated in Fig. 6.14, where the extracted pulse energy (solid line) is plotted versus the stored optical energy. The amplifier output energies lie below the guide line for an optimized amplifier chain performance (second design), which is shown by the dotted line. The large deviations between the two designs result from inadequate matching of the amplifiers in the first design. This is due to the fact that the scaling laws for an amplifier chain were not well established when the ASTERIX III laser was built.

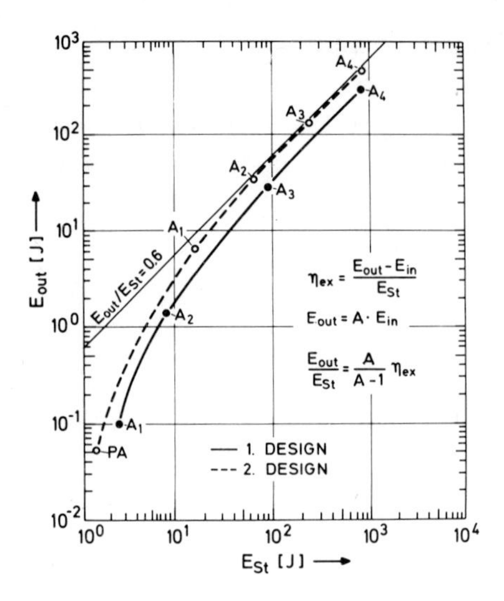

Fig. 6.14. Dependence of the output energy E_{out} on the stored inversion energy E_{St} of the ASTERIX III laser (first and second design). The energy amplification A is different for each amplifier in the first design, whereas in the second design the main amplifiers (A_2,A_3,A_4) have nearly the same amplification ($A \sim 6$)

The average energy extraction efficiency of the first design is $\eta_{ex} = 0.3$ and that of the second was calculated to be of the order of $\eta_{ex} = 0.45$. In the second design, a preamplifier is added and the stored inversion energies of the first, second, and third amplifiers are increased. Furthermore the first amplifier is operated in the double pass mode, described in Sect. 5.1.1. All these measures lead to an enhancement of the input energy densities of the amplifiers and hence to a higher saturation, The output energy of the system is thus expected to rise from 300 to 500 J and the overall efficiency correspondingly from 0.08% to 0.13%.

7. Scalability and Prospects of the Iodine Laser

With the continuing use of the ASTERIX III system for laser plasma experiments, experience in the handling of a large iodine laser is accumulating. In view of the favourable performance of this laser, it is thus appropriate to discuss its scalability to a new generation of large-scale iodine laser systems for research applications (scientific break-even). Such lasers should not only provide higher output energy and power, but also include additional features such as pulse lengths longer than those hitherto obtained (up to several ns) and possibly pulse shaping. Moreover, a better overall efficiency than that realized so far is also desirable. These questions are dealt with in the first two sections of this chapter.

The last section is concerned with the prospective of application of the iodine laser in a fusion power plant, i.e. its possible use as a driver. Here additional requirements have to be met. These include an overall efficiency of a few per cent and a repetition rate in the range of 1 to 10 Hz. The three most effective pumping schemes are analysed with regard to the attainment of higher efficiencies.

7.1 Scalability

In this section the scaling of an iodine laser system to output energies on the order of 100 kJ is discussed. Only present technologies and concepts will be considered.

An energy of this order of magnitude cannot be delivered in a single beam. To restrict the number of arms it will therefore be necessary to put as much energy as possible into one beam. There are, however, some limitations on such a design.

The first concerns the beam diameter. It should not exceed a certain size. Otherwise the optical components become too expensive since costs of these components scale with the cube of the aperture. In addition, the restrictions imposed by the decrease in the appropriate $i\text{-}C_3F_7I$ pressure with increasing beam diameter (which necessarily leads to declining stored energy per unit volume) limit the beam diameter. From our present perspective a diameter of 50 cm therefore seems a reasonable upper limit.

The second restriction arises from limitations on the laser flux imposed by the B integral and from the damage thresholds of optical components or coatings. The B integral limitation plays a role for pulses shorter than 0.5 ns (Sect. 4.1.1). The restrictions originating from damage thresholds lead (according to the recommendations given in Sect. 5.3.3 to limit the maximum beam loading e_m to be one half of the median damage threshold) to the following values of e_m for 1 ns pulses: $e_m \sim 8$ J/cm^2 for polished bare surfaces, $e_m \sim 2.5$-4 J/cm^2 for AR coatings, $e_m \sim 6$ J/cm^2 for graded index AR surfaces (neutral solution processed), $e_m \sim 4.5$-7.5 J/cm^2 for HR coatings and $e_m \sim 2$ J/cm^2 (p polarization) and $e_m \sim 4$ J/cm^2 (s polarization) for thin film polarizers.

Whether the fluence limited beam loading can be obtained depends on the stored inversion energy density e_{st} (J/cm^2) and the extraction efficiency η_{ex}. In an amplifier which can sustain buffer gas pressures of up to 10 bar, the maximum stored energy density will be about 8 J/cm^2 if the small-signal amplification has a value of 100. Provided that the amplifier input energy density is 1 J/cm^2, the extraction efficiency will be $\eta_{ex} = 55\%$ (Sect. 5.1.1). Consequently, the maximum beam loading of the output window is about 5.5 J/cm^2. This value is above the damage threshold of conventional AR coatings and therefore either uncoated windows (tilted or at Brewster's angle) or graded index surfaces have to be used.

Based upon conservative scaling of contemporary laser systems, it can be concluded that a 100 kJ system would be entirely within the range of present technological capabilities. With a pulse length of 1 ns and a beam loading of about 5.5 J/cm^2, such an installation would require 9 beams each having an output diameter of 50 cm. If the pumping time is kept at 10 µs, a reduction of the useful diameter due to the shock wave plays no role at such a large diameter.

The length of the amplifier would be determined by the pumping geometry. With flashlamps placed inside and outside the laser medium, the $i\text{-}C_3F_7I$ pressure could be raised by 30% compared with exclusively external pumping. The active length of the amplifier is then correspondigly reduced and according to (3.13) has a value of $\ell = 20$ m. With an overall efficiency of $\eta_o = 0.3\%$ (Table 7.1), each amplifier would require a capacitor bank energy of 3.6 MJ.

With regard to maintenance and iodide replacement, a significant scaling-up of present installations would be necessary, but no unsurmountable problems are expected. For example, the iodide consumption of a final amplifier would be 90 g of C_3F_7I per shot if photolysis is assumed to be irreversible. However, at an extraction efficiency of 55% the transition is highly saturated and a reduction in medium consumption of at least a factor of two through recombination is anticipated (see Sect. 2.3.3).

Other considerations apply to the addition of options such as a changeable pulse width or a tailored output pulse. As mentioned above, subnanosecond pulses would probably lead to additional limitations imposed by the B integral. However, changing the pulse width in the region of a nanosecond is relatively easy since it can be shown that the output pulse width of an iodine laser amplifier chain is a monotonically increasing function of the input pulse width [7.1].

It would be much more difficult to get a tailored pulse shape since ultrashort pulses and the application of a pulse-stacking device would be needed.

7.2 Efficiency Considerations

The potential for enhancement of the overall efficiency of a laser system is of vital interest for saving costs in the construction of a large-scale research laser, because the costs for the equipment necessary to store and handle the electric energy constitute a large fraction of the total system costs.

It has already been stated in Sect. 5.1 that the overall laser efficiency, (defined as the quotient of the laser pulse energy and the electric energy stored in the capacitor banks) depends on the efficiency of the two main processes, namely pumping and energy extraction. As the details of the energy extraction have already been discussed in Sects. 3.3.2 and 5.1, the following explanations will mainly deal with the pumping process. Its efficiency η_p results from a sequence of internal processes. These processes will be described by the following parameters:

a) First there is the quantum efficiency η_q. Its value is determined by the frequency relation between pumping and laser light.

b) As a fraction of the electric energy is lost in the transmission line between the capacitors and the flashlamps, it is not possible to utilize all of the stored electric energy in the pumping process. The fraction available is specified by the energy transfer factor η_{tr}.

c) The energy transferred to the flashlamps will, to a certain extent, be converted into light emitted in the absorption band of the iodides. This process is determined by the lamp efficiency η_l.

d) Only a fraction of the light emitted by the flashlamps is radiated into the amplifiers. This fraction, which is described by the coupling factor η_c, depends on the geometric arrangement of the flashlamps, their reflectors, and the reflectivity of the reflectors.

e) Not all of the pumping light can be absorbed in the amplifiers, since otherwise the C_3F_7I pressure would be too high and the inversion profile would become too inhomogeneous for pulse amplification. The fraction absorbed is given by the absorption factor η_{ab}.

The pumping efficiency η_p for the stored inversion energy is then: $\eta_p = \eta_q \eta_{tr} \eta_l \eta_c \eta_{ab}$. Not all of the stored inversion energy is available for the extraction process. The volumetric reductions in the active medium caused by the formation of shock waves (Sect. 4.2.1) have to be taken into account. The fraction of the stored inversion energy which can be used for the amplification process is described in the following:

f) Only the amplifier cross-section not obscured by the shock wave can be used for amplification. The fraction available is defined by the area utilization factor K.

g) The losses caused by the shock wave also depend on the length of pumping time. They can be reduced by sending the laser pulse through the amplifier before the pumping process has been fully completed. The energy of the low-intensity tail at the end of the pumping process which is not used is then more than compensated by the gain in useful amplifier cross-sectional area. The fraction of the total pumping energy emitted before the release of the laser is given by the pumping energy utilization factor P.

h) The fraction of energy which will be extracted by the pulse is described by the extraction efficiency η_{ex}. Its value depends on various parameters as outlined in Sect. 3.2.

i) Not all of the energy extracted from an amplifier will propagate to the following one. Absorption takes place in the amplifier decoupling elements. The fraction of the total extracted pulse energy transmitted through the chain is described by the transmission factor $Tr = 1-(E_{out})_{EA}/\sum_{i=1}^{n}(E_{out})_i$ ($(E_{out})_{EA}$ - output energy of the end amplifier).

The product of all the parameters describing the internal processes specifies the overall system efficiency η_o:

$$\eta_o = \eta_q \eta_{tr} \eta_l \eta_c \eta_{ab} K P \eta_{ex} Tr. \tag{7.1}$$

The average values of the energy utilization and transmission factors and of the internal and the overall efficiencies attained at present with the ASTERIX III laser system are listed in Table 7.1 together with projected maximum values of an advanced system having an output energy in the kJ range.

Table 7.1 Efficienies and energy utilization and transmission factors

Specification		ASTERIX III [%]	projected values [%]
Quantum efficiency	η_q	21	21
Electric energy transm. factor	η_{tr}	80	90
Lamp efficiency	η_l	8	8
Coupling factor	η_c	70	75
Absorption factor	η_{ab}	60	75
Area utilization factor	K	65	80
Pumping energy utilization factor	P	80	90
Extraction efficiency	η_{ex}	30	55
Transmission factor	Tr	90	90
Overall efficiency	η_o	0.08	0.30

The ASTERIX III values are derived from measurements and calculations for each individual amplifier stage and then averaged over the chain. The pumping efficiency η_p is obtained by measuring the total stored inversion energy. The value of the extraction efficiency η_{ex} is derived from the measured total stored inversion energy by taking into account the utilization factors for the amplifier cross-section and the pumping time. The relatively low value of the extraction efficiency of η_{ex} = 30% results from the fact that the amplifiers of the ASTERIX III system are not adequately staged and therefore not really saturated.

The maximum efficiency values of an advanced laser system are expected to be obtained for an optimized future flashlamp pumped multi-kJ laser built according to our present knowledge. The maximum values of the internal efficiencies can only be obtained when flashlamps imbedded in the laser medium are additionally employed, and when the laser losses caused by the shock waves are small due to short pumping times and large amplifier cross-sections.

A comparison of the values of the different internal efficiencies in Table 7.1 shows that a substantial increase of the overall efficiency of a photolytically pumped iodine laser can only be expected if one succeeds in raising the lamp efficiency. Although this efficiency has already been doubled for a few shots to a value of $\eta_l = 20\%$ with specially doped xenon gas [7.2], much effort is still necessary to develop efficient, long-lived, high energy flashlamps suitable for practical applications.

These considerations have dealt only with the single-shot efficiency of the laser. However, since in this photolytic laser the laser medium is partially consumed during operation, an additional efficiency originating from the need to regenerate the medium has to be considered. The overall efficiency including the laser medium regeneration is then defined by

$$\eta_o^* = E_l/(E_p + E_r) \tag{7.2}$$

where E_l is the laser pulse energy, E_p the electric pumping energy, and E_r the regeneration energy. According to [7.3] the regeneration efficiency is defined by

$$\eta_r = E_l/E_r \ . \tag{7.3}$$

Using this definition and $\eta_o = E_l/E_p$, (7.2) can be written

$$\eta_o^* = \eta_o \, \eta_r/(\eta_o + \eta_r) \ . \tag{7.4}$$

With $i\text{-}C_3F_7I$ as the laser medium a value of 12% is estimated for η_r in [7.3]. As the maximum value of the overall efficiency is $\eta_o = 0.3\%$, the regeneration of the laser medium introduces only a negligible decrease of the overall efficiency η_o.

7.3 Application Prospects of the Iodine Laser in a Fusion Power Plant

If the iodine laser is to be used as a driver in an inertial confinement fusion power plant, it has to meet two requirements in addition to those needed in a big research laser having an output energy of several hundred kilojoules (as discussed in the previous sections). Firstly, the overall efficiency has to be a few per cent [7.4,5]. Secondly, the repetition rate must be in the range between 1 and 10 Hz. In the following discussion, three pumping schemes envisaged at present as the most effective ones are examined with respect to these two requirements.

First the flashlamp-pumped system is considered. Since the overall efficiency of such a system is below 1% and the flashlamps cannot be expected to take more than 10^6 shots, corresponding to a lifetime of only 1 day at a repetition rate of 10 Hz, it is obvious that this technology is not suited to this kind of application. Further restrictions also arise from the capacitor bank, the lifetime of which will not be much longer than that of the flashlamps, estimated according to the present state of the art.

More interesting in this fusion power plant context is the excitation scheme based on the use of low-pressure mercury lamps. They have an efficiency of more than 20% for converting electric energy into UV light at 254 nm [7.6], which is well within the absorption spectrum of the RI molecules. It therefore seems possible to build laser systems with an overall efficiency close to 1%. However, these Hg lamps have a low power per unit length of only 2 W/cm compared with 3×10^5 W/cm for xenon flashlamps. This disadvantage can be compensated by longer pumping times with an upper limit of a few milliseconds (limited by quenching of I*) and much larger system dimensions [7.7]. For the same output energy the active volume of a Hg--lamp-pumped system has to be roughly 10^3 times greater than that of a xenon-flashlamp-pumped system. Although the Hg lamps and the pertinent electrical network will probably be free of any serious lifetime problems owing to the low loading, the huge dimensions of a several hundred kilojoule system appear to be prohibitive for application as a driver in a fusion power plant.

Another scheme which has been proposed as a candidate for a high efficiency laser fusion driver is chemical pumping of an iodine laser, already discussed in Sect. 2.2.4. This method applies the energy transfer from excited oxygen molecules to the iodine atom [7.8]. The pumping reaction is

$$O_2(^1\Delta) + I(^2P_{3/2}) \rightleftharpoons O_2(^1\Sigma) + I(^2P_{1/2}) \qquad (7.5)$$

The excited oxygen molecule $O_2(^1\Delta)$ can be effectively and cheaply produced by means of chemical generation [7.9]. Unfortunately, the situation is such that the $O_2(^1\Delta)$ concentration has to be 10-20 times larger than the $I(^2P_{1/2})$ concentration in order to achieve an $I(^2P_{1/2})$ lifetime of a few milliseconds. This time is necessary for efficient mixing of the two gases. The main reaction limiting the $I(^2P_{1/2})$ lifetime is

$$I(^2P_{1/2}) + O_2(^1\Delta) \rightarrow I(^2P_{3/2}) + O_2(^1\Sigma) \quad . \tag{7.6}$$

This reaction is a loss process for $O_2(^1\Delta)$ since there is no kinetic pathway allowing energy stored in $O_2(^1\Sigma)$ to be used to excite iodine atoms. The fact that the density of $O_2(^1\Delta)$ is much larger than that of $I(^2P_{1/2})$ means that the energy is almost exclusively stored in the $O_2(^1\Delta)$ molecules rather than in the iodine atoms. Multiple pass techniques have thus to be applied to extract the energy from the amplifier [7.9-11]. A system study of an amplifier based on this scheme has been performed in [7.9]. In the example investigated the initial mixture consists of 130 mbar argon, 0.4 mbar I_2 and 13 mbar O_2 with 80% $O_2(^1\Delta)$, corresponding to 36 J/l stored in the $O_2(^1\Delta)$ molecules at the beginning. It was estimated in [7.9] that from this energy 15 J/l can be extracted in 20 passes by the pulse to be amplified. The time needed to reestablish equilibrium between O_2 and I after one pass is 200 ns. This time interval can be realized by mounting the mirrors at an appropriate distance from the amplifier (L = 33 m).

An amplifier capable of generating an output energy of 100 kJ could be quite compact. With 15 J/l as extractable energy density, the active medium would occupy a cylinder 3 m long and 1.7 m in diameter [7.9]. The output fluence would be 5 J/cm^2. The length-to-diameter ratio is suitable for efficient angle-resolved multiple pass extraction. Such a scheme may be nessessary since large aperture fast optical switches are still in the development stage. The overall efficiency defined as the ratio of the laser output energy over the energy required for chemical regeneration of the starting material is predicted to be 6% [7.9,10]. Even higher values between 10%-15% are estimated for a system with a cooled laser medium [7.11].

Despite these favourable predictions, the realization of such a system seems to be quite difficult. There are still many open questions concerning, for example, the scaling of chemical generators, the extrapolation to higher gas pressures and the lifetime of the gain. Moreover the detailed kinetics, of the chemical iodine laser are still unknown. In view of these uncertainties, it seems at the moment too early to predict that CW chemical pumping will lead to a highly efficient, high power iodine laser.

8. Conclusion

The iodine laser in its present state of development can be considered as a reliable tool for research on laser-produced plasma. Its capability of producing subnanosecond pulses of good beam quality at the TW power level has been demonstrated. Design of a system with energies of approximately 100 kJ with pulse durations ranging from 100 ps to several ns seems to be entirely feasible on the basis of present flashlamp technology and laser design.

There is, however, still room for further improvements in the performance of the iodine laser. On a short term basis the overall efficiency can be increased by a factor of three utilising faster flashlamps, reflectors with $R \geqq 80\%$ and mixtures of n-C_3F_7I and t-C_4F_9I to facilitate a broader UV-absorption linewidth. On a long term basis significant potential exists for further development of excimer (fluorescence and laser) and chemical pumping technologies. The applicability of e-beam- or proton-beam-pumped excimers (KrF or XeCl) as the dissociation sources for large aperture amplifiers is attractive because the short pumping time (~ 30 ns) diminishes the problem of amplifier coupling, thereby allowing for higher stored energy densities. Chemical pumping offers the advantages of compactness, high efficiency and high repetition rate. Problems, however, arise with the conversion of stored chemical energy into laser light. In this area future research effort has to be concentrated.

Besides this evaluation of the development potential of the iodine laser it is also instructive to compare its performance with those of the Nd glass and CO_2 lasers, which all meet the requirements imposed by fusion experiments.

An important criterion for any big research laser is the capital cost per joule of focusible energy. For Nd glass and iodine an evaluation of this figure was made on the basis of a comparison of the ARGUS (LLL) and ASTERIX III systems [8.1]. It turned out that for pulse lengths smaller than about 2 ns, the cost situation is in favour of iodine. For longer pulses there is at present no appreciable cost difference between the two laser systems. Unfortunately, owing to the lack of appropriate data, no equivalent study could be made for the CO_2 laser.

Besides these cost considerations, other criteria of similar importance should also be taken into account. These refer to the repetition rate, the maintenance effort and the structural complexity and the corresponding sensitivity of a system with respect to misfiring and possible damage of laser components. Since the iodine and CO_2 lasers, on the one hand, have a considerably smaller number of components and optical surfaces than a Nd glass laser for comparable output energy and power and since, on the other hand, the working medium of iodine and CO_2 is a gas, these two lasers possess advantages over the Nd laser. Although the technologies of the iodine and CO_2 lasers are rather different from each other, there are no major differences between them regarding their performance in view of the aforementioned criteria. The shorter wavelength is a significant advantage for the iodine laser, while the high efficiency (~2%) of the CO_2 laser favours its use in a pilot fusion test reactor.

Since laser plasma research is ultimately directed towards a laser fusion power plant, promising high-power lasers therefore need to be examined in view of their possible application as a driver in a fusion power station. Here additional requirements arise which can be summarized as follows: megajoule pulses with durations of up to a few nanoseconds, a repetition rate between 1 and 10 Hz and an overall efficiency of the laser of a few per cent.

While even megajoule pulse energies are within the scope of present technology of the flashlamp-pumped iodine laser, it is clear that the required repetition rate and overall efficiency cannot be attained by this pumping scheme. These requirements can only be met by entirely different pumping methods such as chemical or direct electrical pumping. From the present state of the art, chemical pumping appears to be the most promising of the two. There is a good chance that excitation schemes can be found which allow for higher atomic iodine inversion densities than is the case with the O_2/I_2 system. This facilitates the energy extraction problem considerably and leads to relatively simple laser configurations. These are necessary in view of the many requirements which have to be fulfilled simultaneously.

References

Chapter 1

1.1 J.V.V. Kasper, G.C. Pimentel: Appl. Phys. Lett. 5, 231 (1964)
1.2 D. Porret, C.F. Goodeve: Proc. R. Soc. London A165, 31 (1938)
1.3 J.V.V. Kasper, J.H. Parker, G.C. Pimemtel: Phys. Rev. Lett. 14, 352 (1965): J. Chem. Phys. 43, 1827 (1965)
1.4 M.A. Pollack: Appl. Phys. Lett. 8, 36 (1966)
1.5 R.J. Donovan, D. Hussain: Chem. Soc. London Ann.Rep. A68, 148 (1971)
1.6 A.J. DeMaria, C.J. Ultee: Appl. Phys. Lett. 9, 67 (1966)
1.7 C.M. Ferrar: Appl. Phys. Lett. 12, 381 (1968)
1.8 D.W. Gregg, R.E. Kidder, C.V. Dobler: Appl. Phys. Lett. 13, 297 (1968)
1.9 P. Gensel, K. Hohla, K.L. Kompa: Appl. Phys. Lett. 18, 48 (1971)
1.10 K. Hohla: Report IPP IV/33, Max-Planck-Institut für Plasmaphysik (1971)
1.11 V.S. Zuev, V.A. Katulin, V. Yu. Nosach, O. Yu. Nosach: Sov. Phys. JETP 35, 870 (1972)
1.12 F.T. Aldridge: Appl. Phys. Lett. 22, 180 (1973)
1.13 E.A. Yukov: Sov. J. Quantum Electron. 3, 117 (1973)
1.14 F.T. Aldridge: IEEE J.Quantum Electron. QE-11, 215 (1975)
1.15 W. Fuss, K. Hohla: Z. Naturforsch. A31, 569 (1976)
1.16 T.D. Patrick, R.E. Palmer: J. Chem. Phys. 62, 3350 (1975)
1.17 K. Hohla, P. Gensel, K.L. Kompa: "Photochemical Iodine Laser - A High-Power Gas Laser", in *Laser Interaction and Related Plasma Phenomena*, ed. by J. Schwarz, H. Hora (Plenum, New York 1972) Vol. 2, pp. 61-66
1.18 N.G. Basov, L.E. Golubev, V.S. Zuev, V.A. Katulin, V.N. Netemin, V.Y. Nosach, O.Y. Nosach, A.L. Petrov: Sov. J. Quantum Electron. 3, 524 (1974)
1.19 K. Hohla, K.L. Kompa: IEEE J. Quantum Electron. QE-8, 198 (1972)
1.20 G. Brederlow, K.J. Witte, E. Fill, K. Hohla, R. Volk: IEEE J. Quantum Electron. QE-12, 152 (1976)
1.21 N.G. Basov, V.S. Zuev: Nuovo Cimento 31B, 129 (1976)
1.22 R.E. Palmer, T.D. Padrick, M.A. Palmer: Opt. Quantum Electron 11, 61 (1978)
1.23 S.B. Kormer: Izv. Akad. Nauk SSSR Ser. Fiz. 44, 2002 (1980)
1.24 K. Eidmann, G. Brederlow, R. Brodmann, R. Petsch, R. Sigel, G. Tsakiris, R. Volk, S. Witkowski: Report PLF 4, Projektgruppe für Laserforschung (1978)
1.25 J.F. Holzwarth, A. Schmidt, H. Wolf, R. Volk: J. Chem. Phys. 81, 2300 (1977)
1.26 T.L. Andreva, G.N. Binch, I.I. Sobelman, V.N. Sorokin, I.I. Struk: Sov. J. Quantum Electron. 7, 1230 (1977)
1.27 K.J. Witte, P. Burkhard, H.R. Lüthi: Opt. Commun. 28, 202 (1979)
1.28 R.J. Richardson, C.E. Wiswall: Appl. Phys. Lett. 35, 138 (1979)

Chapter 2

2.1 R.H. Garstang: J. Res. Nat. Bur. Stand. A68, 61 (1964)
2.2 D.E. O'Brien, J.R. Bowen: J. Appl. Phys. 40, 4769 (1969)
2.3 R.J. Donovan, D. Hussain: Chem. Soc. London Ann. Rep. A68, 148 (1971)
2.4 V.S. Zuev, V.A. Katulin, V. Yu. Nosach, O. Yu. Nosach: Sov. Phys. JETP 35, 870 (1972)
2.5 F.J. Comes, S. Piontek: Chem. Phys. Lett. 42, 558 (1976)
2.6 M. Galanti, W. Thieme, K.J. Witte: IEEE J. Quantum Electron. QE-17, 1817 (1981)
2.7 L.S. Ershov, V. Yu. Zalesskii: Sov. J. Quantum Electron. 8, 649 (1978)
2.8 E. Gerck, E. Fill: Opt. Lett. 7, 25 (1981)
2.9 V. Jaccarino, J.G. King, R.A. Satten, H.H. Stroke: Phys. Rev. 94, 1798 (1954)
2.10 E. Luc-König, C. Morillon, J. Verges: Phys. Scr. 12, 199 (1975)
2.11 Engleman, R.A. Keller, B.A. Palmer: Appl. Opt. 19, 2767 (1981)
2.12 V.A. Aleekseev, T.L. Andreeva, V.N. Volkov, E.A. Yukov: Sov. Phys. JETP 36, 238 (1973)
2.13 E.A. Yukov: Sov. J. Quantum Electron. 3, 117 (1973)
2.14 E.S. Mukhtar, H.J. Baker, T.A. King: Opt. Commun. 19, 193 (1976)
E.S. Mukhtar, H.J. Baker, T.A. King: Opt. Commun. 24, 167 (1978)
2.15 T.D. Padrick, E.A. Palmer: J. Chem. Phys. 62, 3350 (1975)
2.16 W. Fuss, K. Hohla: IPP-Report IV/67 (1974); Z. Naturf. 31a, 569 (1976)
2.17 F.T. Aldridge: Appl. Phys. Lett. 22, 180 (1973)
2.18 F.T. Aldridge: IEEE J. Quantum Electr. QE-11, 215 (1975)
2.19 V.I. Babkin, S.N. Kuznetsova, A.I. Maslov: Sov. J. Quantum Electron. 8, 825 (1978)
2.20 H.J. Baker, T.A. King: J. Phys. D 9, 2433 (1976)
2.21 V. Yu. Zalesskii, S.S. Polikarpov: Sov. J. Quantum Electr. 5, 826 (1975)
2.22 H.J. Baker, T.A. King: J. Phys. D 8, 609 (1975)
2.23 I.M. Belousova, B.D. Bobrov, V.M. Kiselev, and V.N. Kurzenkov: Sov. J. Quantum Electr. 4, 767 (1974)
2.24 D.W. Gregg, R.E. Kidder, C.V. Dobler: Appl. Phys. Lett. 13, 297 (1968)
2.25 I.M. Belousova, B.D. Bobrov, V.M. Kiselev, V.N. Kurzenkov, P.I. Krepostnov: Sov. Phys. JETP 38, 258 (1974)
2.26 V.A. Katulin, V. Yu. Nosach, A.L. Petrov: Sov. J. Quantum Electr. 8, 380 (1978)
2.27 V.M. Kiselev, B.D. Bobrov, A.S. Grenishin, T.N. Kotlikova: Sov. J. Quantum Electron. 8, 181 (1978)
2.28 E.E. Fill, W.H. Thieme, R. Volk: J. Phys. D 12, 41 (1979)
2.29 I.M. Belousova, B.D. Bobrov, V.M. Kiselev, V.N. Kurzenkov, P.I. Krepostnov: Opt. Spectrosc. 37, 20 (1974)
2.30 N.M. Gibbs, G.G. Churchill, T.R. Marshall, J.E. Papp, E.A. Franz: Phys. Rev. Lett. 25, 263 (1970);
A. Gallagher: Phys. Rev. 157, 68 (1975)
2.31 V.A. Katulin, V. Yu. Nosach, A.L. Petrov: Sov. J. Quantum Electron. 9, 169 (1979)
2.32 W. Thieme, E. Fill: J. Phys. D 12, 2031 (1979)
2.33 W. Thieme, E. Fill: Opt. Commun. 36, 361 (1981)
2.34 D.J. Benard, W.E. McDermott, N.R. Pchelkin, R.R. Bousek: Appl. Phys. Lett. 34, 40 (1979)
2.35 D. Porret, C.F. Goodeve: Proc. R. Soc. London A31, 165 (1938)
2.36 J.V.V. Kasper, G.C. Pimentel: Appl. Phys. Lett. 5, 231 (1964)

2.37 T.L. Andreeva, V.A. Dudkin, V.I. Malyshev, G.C. Mikhailov, V.N. Sorokin, L.A. Novikova: Sov. Phys. JETP 22, 969 (1066)
2.38 E. Gerck: MPQ Rep. No. 58 (1982), Max-Planck-Institut für Quantenoptik, 8046 Garching, FRG
2.39 L.G. Karpov, A.M. Pravilov, F.I. Vilesov: Sov. J. Quantum Electron. 7, 497 (1977)
2.40 G.N. Birich, G.I. Drozd, V.N. Sorokin, I.I. Struk: JETP Lett. 19, 27 (1974)
2.41 H. Hoffmann, St. R. Leone: J. Chem. Phys. 69, 3819 (1978)
2.42 S.J. Davis: Appl. Phys. Lett. 32, 656 (1978)
2.43 H. Pummer, J. Eggleston, W.V. Bishel, C.K. Rhodes: Appl. Phys. Lett. 32, 427 (1978)
2.44 T.D. Padrick: Res. Progr. Rep. SAND 78-0811, Sandia Laboratories, 39 (1978)
2.45 J.F. Holzrichter, H.A. Pumberton, N. Dobeck, T. Douich: LLL Rep. UCRL-77696; CLEA, San Diego 1976
2.46 N.J. Dobeck, J.F. Holzrichter, H.A. Pumberton: LLL Rep. UCRL-76345; Also: IEEE/OSA Conf. Washington D.C. 1975
2.47 T. Nakamura: IPP Internal Report (1973), Max-Planck-Institut für Plasmaphysik, 8046 Garching, FRG
2.48 K. Hohla: In *High Power Lasers and Applications*, ed. by K. Kompa, H. Walther, Springer Series in Optical Sciences, Vol. 9 (Springer, Berlin, Heidelberg, New York 1978) p. 124
2.49 A.S. Antonov: Sov. Tech. Phys. Lett. 4, 459 (1978)
2.50 M.A. Gusinov: Opt. Commun. 15, 190 (1975)
2.51 R.E. Palmer: Res. Progr. Rep. SAND 78-0811, Sandia Laboratories, p. 33 (1978); Res. Progr. Rep. SAND 78-2306, Sandia Laboratories, p. 31 (1978)
2.52 A.F. Alexandrov, A.A. Rukhadse: Sov. Phys. Usp. 17, 44 (1974)
2.53 N.G. Basov, V.S. Zuev, V.A. Katulin, A. Yu. Lyubchenko, V. Yu. Nosach, A.L. Petrov: Kvantovaya Elektron. 6, 311 (1979)
2.54 N.G. Basov, V.S. Zuev: Nuovo Cimento 31B, 129 (1976)
2.55 R.E. Beverly, R.H. Barnes, C.E. Moeller: Appl. Opt. 16, 1572 (1977)
2.56 P. Gensel, K.L. Kompa, J. Wanner: Chem. Phys. Lett. 7, 583 (1970)
2.57 R.E. Beverly, R.H. Barnes, L. Yin: Opt. Commun. 14, 412 (1975)
2.58 W.T. Silfvast, L.H. Szeto, O.R. Wood II: Appl. Phys. Lett. 25, 593 (1974)
2.59 C.K. Rhodes (ed.): *Excimer Lasers*, Topics in Applied Physics, Vol. 30 (Springer, Berlin, Heidelberg, New York 1979)
2.60 W.F. Krupke, E.V. George: LLL-Rep. UCRL-77523 (1976)
2.61 J.C. Swingle, C.E. Turner, J.R. Murray, E.V. George, W.F. Krupke: Appl. Phys. Lett. 28, 387 (1976)
2.62 E. Fill, W. Skrlac, K.J. Witte: Opt. Commun. 37, 123 (1982)
2.63 V. Yu. Zalesskii; Sov. Phys. JETP 40, 14 (1975)
2.64 V. Yu. Zalesskii, M.G. Ivanov: Sov. J. Quantum Electron. 5, 156 (1975); Sov. J. Quantum Electron. 5, 1396 (1975)
2.65 L.D. Pleasance, L.A. Weaver: Appl. Phys. Lett. 27, 407 (1975)
2.66 M.C. Wong, R.E. Beverly III: Opt. Commun. 20, 19 (1977)
2.67 R.E. Beverly III, M.C. Wong: Opt. Commun. 20, 23 (1977)
2.68 W.E. McDermott, N.R. Pchelkin, D.J. Benard, R.R. Bousek: Appl. Phys. Lett. 32, 469 (1978)
2.69 R.J. Richardson, C.E. Wiswall: Appl. Phys. Lett. 35, 138 (1979)
2.70 G.N. Hays, G.A. Fisk: IEEE J. Quantum Electron. QE-17, 1823, (1981)
2.71 R.G. Derwent, B.A. Thrush: Faraday Discuss. Chem. Soc. 53, 162 (1972)
2.72 R.G. Avilés, D.F. Muller, P.L. Houston: Appl. Phys. Lett. 37, 358 (1980)
2.73 D.F. Muller, R.H. Young, P.L. Houston, J.R. Wiesenfeld: Appl. Phys. Lett. 38, 404 (1981)

2.74 R.F. Heidner: 3rd Tech. Digest Topical Meeting Infrared Lasers, Los Angeles, CA, Dec. 3-5, (1980)
2.75 G.E. Busch: IEEE J. Quantum Electron. QE-17, 1128, (1981)
2.76 R. Donohue, J.R. Wiesenfeld: Chem. Phys. Lett. 33, 176 (1975)
2.77 R. Donohue, J.R. Wiesenfeld: J. Chem. Phys. 63, 3130 (1975)
2.78 A.M. Pravilov: Sov. J. Quantum Electron. 11, 847 (1981)
2.79 R.J. Donovan, F.G.M. Hathorn, D. Husain: Trans. Faraday Soc. 64, 3192 (1968)
2.80 T.L. Andreeva, V.A. Dudkin, V.I. Malyshev, G.C. Mikhailov, V.N. Sorokin, L.A. Novikova: Sov. Phys. JETP 22, 969 (1966)
2.81 V. Yu. Zalesskii, T.I. Krupenikova: Opt. Spectrosc. USSR, 30, 439 (1971)
2.82 R.J. Donovan, C. Fotakis: I. Chem. Phys. 61, 2169 (1974)
2.83 S.V. Kuznetsova, A.I. Maslov: Sov. J. Quantum Electron. 3, 468 (1974)
2.84 C.C. Davis, R.J. Pirkle, R.A. McFarlane, G.J. Wolga: IEEE J. Quantum Electron. QE-12, 334 (1976)
2.85 K. Hohla, K.L. Kompa: In *Handbook of Chemical Lasers*, ed. by R.W. Gross & J.F. Bott, (John Wiley & Sons, New York 1976) pp. 667-701
2.86 L.S. Ershov, V. Yu. Zalesskii, V.N. Sokolov: Sov. J. Quantum Electron. 8, 494 (1978)
2.87 V.S. Ivanov, A.S. Kozlov, A.M. Pravilov, E.P. Smirnov: Sov. J. Quantum Electron. 10, 566 (1980)
2.88 A.M. Pravilov, A.S. Kozlov, V.I. Vilesov: Sov. J. Quantum Electron. 8, 666 (1978)
2.89 K.J. Witte: Opt. Commun. 37, 293 (1981)
2.90 W. Fuss, K. Hohla: Opt. Commun. 18, 427 (1976)
2.91 K.J. Witte: To be published
2.92 A.J. DeMaria, C.J. Ultzee: Appl. Phys. Lett. 9, 67 (1966)
2.93 T.L. Andreeva, V.I. Malyshev, A.I. Maslov, I.I. Sobelman, V.N. Sorokin: Sov. Phys. JETP Lett. 10, 271 (1969)
2.94 T.L. Andreeva, S.V. Kuznetsova, A.I. Maslov, I.I. Sobelman, V.N. Sorokin: Sov. Phys. JETP Lett. 13, 449 (1971)
2.95 P. Gensel, K. Hohla, K. Kompa: Appl. Phys. Lett. 18, 48 (1971)
2.96 K. Hohla, K.L. Kompa: Z. Naturforsch. 27a, 938 (1972)
2.97 K. Hohla, K.L. Kompa: Chem. Phys. Lett. 14, 445 (1972)
2.98 V. Yu. Zalesskii: Sov. Phys. JETP 34, 474 (1972)
2.99 D.H. Burde, R. McFarlane, J.R. Wiesenfeld: Chem. Phys. Lett. 32, 296 (1975)
2.100 G.N. Vinukurov, V. Yu. Zalesskii: Sov. J. Quantum Electron. 8, 1191 (1978)
2.101 I. Arnold, F.J. Comes, S. Piontek: Chem. Phys. 9, 237 (1975)
2.102 D.H. Burde, R.A. McFarlane: J. Chem. Phys. 64, 1850 (1976)
2.103 J.C. Amphlett, E. Whittle: Trans. Faraday Soc. 63, 2695 (1967)
2.104 E. Rabinovitch, W.C. Wood: Trans. Faraday Soc. 32, 540 (1936)
2.105 J. Tellinghuisen: J. Chem. Phys. 58, 2821 (1973)
2.106 M.A. Pollack: Appl. Phys. Lett. 8, 36 (1966)
2.107 D.E. O'Brien, J.R. Bowen: J. Appl. Phys. 40, 4767 (1969)
2.108 D.E. O'Brien, J.R. Bowen: J. Appl. Phys. 42, 1010 (1971)
2.109 V.Y. Zalesskii, A.A. Venediktov: Sov. Phys. JETP 28, 1104 (1969)
2.110 T.L. Andreeva, S.V. Kuznetsova, A.I. Maslov, I.I. Sobelman, V.N. Sorokin: JETP Lett. 13, 449 (1971)
2.111 V. Yu. Zalesskii: Sov. Phys. JETP 34, 474 (1972)
2.112 K. Hohla, K.L. Kompa: Z. Naturforsch. 27a, 938 (1972)
2.113 R.D. Franklin: Tech. Rep. ARL 73-0071; Wright Patterson Air Force Base, Dayton, Ohio, April 1973
2.114 C. Turner, N.L. Rapagnani: Semiannual Report UCRL 50021-73-1, Lawrence Livermore Lab., Jan. - June (1973)
2.115 C. Turner, N.L. Rapagnani: Rep. UCID - 16935 Lawrence Livermore Lab., (1974)

2.116 R.F. Beverley III: Opt. Commun. 15, 204 (1975)
2.117 E.V. Archipova, B.L. Borovich, A.K. Zapolskii: Sov. J. Quantum Electron. 6, 686 (1976)
2.118 E.V. Archipova, B.L. Borovich, A.K. Zapolskii: Sov. J. Quantum Electron. 6, 691 (1976)
2.119 G.A. Fisk: Rep. SAND 77-0880, Sandia Laboratories (1977)
2.120 K.H. Stephan, F.J. Comes: Chem. Phys. Lett. 65, 251 (1979)
2.121 F.J. Comes: Private Communication
2.122 S.L. Dobychin, L.D. Mikhiev, A.B. Pavlov, V.B. Fabanov, M.A. Khodakovsky: Kvantovaya Elektron. 5, 2461 (1978)
2.123 F.J. Comes, S. Pointek: Chem. Phys. Lett. 58, 616 (1978)
2.124 V. Yu. Zalesskii, L.S. Ershov, A.M. Kokushkin, S.S. Polikarpov: Sov. J. Quantum Electron. 11, 498 (1981)
2.125 R.J. Donovan, D. Husain: Chem. Soc. London, Annual Rep. A68, 148 (1971); also in *Advances in Photochemistry 9*, ed. by J.N. Pitts, G.S. Hammond, W.A. Noves (Wiley-Interscience, New York, 1971) p. 45
2.126 J.J. Deakin, D. Hussain: J. Chem. Soc. Faraday II 68, 1603 (1972)
2.127 S.V. Kusnetsova, A.I. Maslov: Sov. J. Quantum Electron. 8, 906 (1978)
2.128 G. Burns, R.J. LeRoy, D.J. Morriss, J.A. Blake: Proc. R. Soc. London A316, 81 (1970)
2.129 J.A. Blake, G. Burns: J. Chem. Phys. 54, 1480 (1971)
2.130 K.E. Russel, J. Simmons: Proc. R. Soc. London A217 (1953)
2.131 B.V. Alekhin, V.V. Borovkov, A. Ya. Brodskii, B.V. Lazhintsev, V.A. Nor-Arevyan, L.Y. Sukhanov: Sov. J. Quantum Electron. 10, 872 (1980)
2.132 V.S. Zuev, V.N. Netemin, O. Yu. Nosach: Sov. J. Quantum Electron. 9, 522 (1979)
2.133 K.J. Witte: J. Phys. D 12, 9 (1979)
2.134 H.M. Wassermann (ed.): *Singlet Oxygen*, Organic Chemistry, Vol. 40 (Academic Press, New York, San Francisco, London 1979) pp. 43-48

Chapter 3

3.1 C.M. Ferrar: Appl. Phys. Lett. 12, 381 (1968)
3.2 D.W. Gregg, R.E. Kidder, C.V. Dobler: Appl. Phys. Lett. 13, 297 (1968)
3.3 I.M. Belousova, B.D. Bobrov, V.M. Kiselev, V.N. Kurzenkov: Sov. J. Quantum Electron 4, 767 (1974)
3.4 G.F. Kozlov, E.F. Stapitskii: Sov. Phys. Tech. Phys. 20, 226 (1975)
3.5 S. Ishii, B. Ahlborn, F.L. Curzon: Appl. Phys. Lett. 27, 118 (1975)
3.6 E. Fill, W. Skrlac, K.J. Witte: Opt. Commun. 37, 123 (1981)
3.7 N.G. Basov, V.S. Zuev: Nuovo Cimento 31B, 129 (1976)
3.8 K. Hohla: Laser Electron Opt. 4, 29 (1972)
3.9 A.E. Siegman, D.J. Kuizenga: Optoelectronics 6, 43 (1974)
3.10 D.J. Kuizenga, D.W. Phillion, T. Land, A.E. Siegman: Opt. Commun. 9, 221 (1972)
3.11 G.C. Guyot, J.C. Farcy, H. Guillet: Rev. Phys. Appl. 12, 1789 (1977)
3.12 K. Hohla, W. Fuss, R. Volk, K.J. Witte: Opt. Commun. 13, 114 (1975)
3.13 R.E. Palmer, T.D. Padrick, M.A. Palmer: Opt. Quantum Electron QE-11, 61 (1979)
3.14 H.J. Baker, T.A. King: Opt. Commun. 18, 21 (1976)
3.15 H.J. Baker, T.A. King: J. Phys., E9, 287 (1976)

3.16 G.T. Schappert, M.J. Herbst: Appl. Phys. Lett. 26, 314 (1975)
3.17 E.D. Jones, M.A. Palmer, F.R. Franklin: Report SAND 75-6052, Sandia Laboratories (1975)
3.18 J.C. Farcy, D. Beaupère, O. de Witte: C.R. Acad. Sci., 284B, 467 (1979)
3.19 E. Fill, K. Hohla: Opt. Commun. 18. 431 (1976)
3.20 K.H. Drexhage, G.A. Reynolds: Opt. Commun. 10, 18 (1974)
3.21 R.W. Eason, R.C. Greenhow, D.M. Goddall, J. Holzwarth: Opt. Commun. 32, 113 (1980)
3.22 M.G. Galpern, V.A. Gorbachev, V.A. Katulin, O.L. Lebedev, E.A. Lukyanets, N.G. Mekhryakova, V.M. Mizin, V.Yu. Nosach, A.L. Petrov, G.G. Semenovkaya: Sov. J. Quantum Electron 5, 1384 (1975)
3.23 V.T. Mueller-Westerhoff: Private communication, IBM Laboratories, San Jose, CA
3.24 K.J. Witte, E. Fill, G. Brederlow, H. Baumhacker, R. Volk: IEEE J. Quantum Electron QE-17, 1809 (1981)
3.25 E. Yablonovitch, J. Goldhar: Appl. Phys. Lett. 25, 580 (1979)
3.26 E. Fill, K. Hohla, G. Schappert: Opt. Commun. 18, 217 (1976)
3.27 E. Fill, K. Hohla, G. Schappert, R. Volk: Appl. Phys. Lett. 29, 805 (1976)
3.28 H.E. Bennet, A.J. Glass, A.H. Guenther, B.E. Newnam (eds.): "Laser induced damage in optical materials", in Natl. Bur. Stand. Spec. Publ.620 and previous volumes (1980)
3.29 W.H. Lowdermilk, D. Milam: IEEE J. Quantum Electron. QE-17, 1888 (1981)
3.30 G. Brederlow, R. Brodmann, K. Eidmann, H. Krause, M. Nippus, R. Petsch, R. Volk, S. Witkowski, K.J. Witte: Report PLF 5, Projektgruppe für Laserforschung (1979)
3.31 J.C. Farcy, M. Huguet, V. Pugliese, J.C. Guyot: Proceedings of 11th Int. Quantum Electron. Conf., Boston, June 1980, paper S 7
3.32 P.G. Kryukov, V.S. Letokhov: Sov. Phys. Usp., 12, 641 (1970)
3.33 A. Iscevgi, W.E. Lamb jr.: Phys. Rev. 185, 517 (1968)
3.34 M.E. Riley, T.D. Padrick, R.E. Palmer: IEEE J. Quantum Electron. QE-15, 178 (1979)
3.35 P.V. Avizonis, F.L. Grotbeck, J. Appl. Phys. 37, 687 (1966)
3.36 W. Fuss, K. Hohla: Z. Naturforsch. A31, 569 (1976)
3.37 H.J. Baker, T.A. King: J. Phys. D9, 2433 (1976)
3.38 M. Nippus: Report PLF 17, Projektgruppe für Laserforschung (1979)
3.39 N. Skribanowitz, B. Kopainsky: Appl. Phys. Lett. 27, 490 (1975)
3.40 J.N. Olsen: J. Appl. Phys. 47, 5360 (1976)
3.41 H. Saito, T. Uchiyama, T. Fujioka: IEEE J. Quantum Electron. QE-14, 302 (1978)
3.42 T. Uchiyama, K.J. Witte: IEEE J. Quantum Electron. QE-18, 885 (1982)

Chapter 4

4.1 J.F. Ward, G.H.C. New: Phys. Rev. 185, 57 (1969)
4.2 D. Eimerl: LLL Annual Report UCRL-50021-78, Vol. 2, Chap. 7, pp. 99-101 (1978)
4.3 A.D. Buckingham, D.A. Dunmur: Trans. Faraday Soc. 64, 1776 (1968); A.D. Buckingham, B.J. Orr: Trans. Faraday Soc. 65, 673 (1969)
4.4 J.F. Ward, I.J. Bigio: Phys. Rev. A11, 60 (1975)
4.5 I.L. Fabelinskii: *Molecular Scattering of Light* (Plenum, New York 1968) p. 555
4.6 D. Milam, M.J. Weber: J. Appl. Phys. 47, 2497 (1976)
4.7 Ch. C. Wang: Phys. Rev. 152, 149 (1966)

4.8 Ch. C. Wang: Phys. Rev. B2, 2045 (1970)
4.9 R.W. Hellwarth: Progress Quantum Electron. 5, Part I (1977)
4.10 D.C. Brown: *High-Peak-Power Nd:Glass Laser Systems*, Springer Series in Optical Sciences, Vol. 25 (Springer, Berlin, Heidelberg, New York 1981)
4.11 J.T. Hunt, J.A. Glaze, W.W. Simmons, P.A. Renard: Appl. Opt. 17, 2053 (1978)
4.12 LLL Annual Report UCRL-50021-76
4.13 J.G. Guyot, A. Bettinguer, D. Auric: Congrés National de Physique des Plasmas, Colloque "Moyens Technique de la Fusion", Paris, 6-10 Dec. 1976
4.14 G. Brederlow, R. Brodmann, K. Eidmann, H. Krause, M. Nippus, R. Petsch, R. Volk, S. Witkowski, K.J. Witte: Report PLF 5, Projektgruppe für Laserforschung, 8046 Garching/FRG (1979)
4.15 L.A. Schlie: J. Opt. Soc. Am. 71, 1080 (1981)
4.16 M.E. Riley, T.D. Patrick, R.E. Palmer: IEEE J. Quantum Electron. QE-15, 178 (1979)
4.17 K. Drühl: J. Chem. Phys. 75, 5579 (1981)
4.18 B.V. Alekhin, V.V. Borovkov, A. Ya. Brodskii, B.V. Lazhintsev, V.A. Nor-Arevyan, L.V. Sukhanov: Sov. J. Quantum Electron. 10, 872 (1980)
4.19 I.E. Gobulev, V.S. Zuev, V.A. Katulin, V.Yu. Nosach, O. Yu. Nosach: Sov. J. Quantum Electron. 3, 464 (1974)
4.20 K.J. Witte: J. Phys. D 12, 9 (1979)
4.21 I.M. Belousova, O.B. Danilov, I.A. Sinitsina, V.V. Spiridonov: Sov. Phys. JETP 31, 791 (1970)
4.22 K. Hohla, K.L. Kompa: Z. Naturforsch. 27a, 938 (1972)
4.23 O.B. Danilov, N.A. Novoselov, V.V. Spiridonov: Opt. Spectrosc. 39, 382 (1975)
4.24 O.B. Danilov, N.A. Novoselov, V.V. Spridonov, N.P. Trofimov: Opt. Spectrosc. 41, 68 (1976)
4.25 T.D. Padrick, R.E. Palmer: J. Appl. Phys. 47, 5109 (1976)
4.26 V.A. Katulin, V.Yu. Nosach, A.L. Petrov: Sov. J. Quantum Electron. 9, 169 (1979)
4.27 G. Brederlow, K.J. Witte, E. Fill, K. Hohla, R. Volk: IEEE J. Quantum Electron. QE-12, 152 (1976)
4.28 N.G. Basov, V.S. Zuev, V.A. Katulin, A. Yu. Lyubchenko, V.Yu. Nosach, A.L. Petrov: Sov. J. Quantum Electron. 9, 174 (1979)
4.29 S.B. Kormer: Izv. Akad. Nauk SSSR Ser. Fiz. 44, 2002 (1980)
4.30 G.N. Vinukurov, V.Yu. Zalesskii: Sov. J. Quantum Electron. 8, 1191 (1978)
4.31 H.J. Baker, T.A. King: IEEE J. Quantum Electron. QE-17, 1828 (1981)
4.32 J.C. Farcy, M. Huguet, V. Pugliese, J.C. Guyot: Int. Quantum Electron. 11th Conf., 23-26 June, 1980, Boston, p. 653
4.33 N.G. Basov, V.S. Zuev: Nuovo Cimento B31, 129 (1976)
4.34 V.A. Katulin, V.Yu. Nosach, A.L. Petrov: Sov. J. Quantum Electron. 9, 169 (1979)
4.35 L.G. Karpov, A.M. Pravilov, F.I. Vilesov: Kvantovaya Elektronika 4, 889 (1977)
4.36 V.S. Zuev, K.N. Netemin, O.Yu. Nosach: Sov. J. Quantum Electron. 9, 522 (1979)
4.37 B.V. Alekhin, V.V. Borovkov, B.V. Lazhintsev, V.A. Nor-Arevyan, L.V. Sukhanov, V.A. Ustinenko: Sov. J. Quantum Electron 9, 1148 (1979)
4.38 V.V. Likhanskii, A.P. Napartovich: Sov. J. Quantum Electron. 11, 384 (1981)
4.39 N.G. Basov, V.S. Zuev, O.Yu. Nosach, E.P. Orlov: Sov. J. Quantum Electron. 10, 1527 (1980)
4.40 V.S. Zuev, E.P. Orlov: Sov. J. Quantum Electron 11, 1191 (1981)
4.41 V.S. Zuev, E.P. Orlov: Sov. J. Quantum Electron 11, 1197 (1981)

4.42 G.W. Sutton: AIAA J. 7, 1737 (1969)
4.43 J.C. Cummings, R.E. Palmer, D.P. Aeschliman: Opt. Commun. 27, 455 (1978)
4.44 M. Nippus: PLF Report 17, Projektgruppe für Laserforschung, 8046 Garching / FRG (1979)
4.45 H. Tennekes, J.L. Lumley: *A First Course in Turbulence* (MIT Press, Cambridge, MA 1972)
4.46 G. Bauer: Z. Phys. Chem. A174, 435 (1935)

Chapter 5

5.1 W.F. Hagen: Report MPQ 52, Max-Planck-Institut für Quantenoptik (1981)
5.2 W.H. Lowdermilk, D. Milam: IEEE J. Quantum Electron. QE-17, 1888 (1981)
5.3 T.D. Padrick, R.E. Palmer: J. Appl. Phys. 47, 5109 (1976)
5.4 L.G. Karpov, A.M. Pravilov, F.I. Vilesov: Sov. J. Quantum Electron 7, 497 (1977)
5.5 W. Fuss, K. Hohla: Opt. Commun. 18, 427 (1976)
5.6 H.J. Baker, T.A. King: J. Phys. D 14, 1367 (1981)
5.7 L.K. Gavrilina, V.A. Katulin, N.N. Korzhavina, Yu. S. Leonov, Yu.I. Morozov, V.Yu. Nosach, A.L. Petrov: Sov. J. Quantum Electron. 9, 874 (1979)
5.8 M.A. Gusinow: IEEE J. Quantum Electron. QE-11, 929 (1975)
5.9 Annual Progress Report on Laser Fusion Programm, Institute of Laser Engineering, Osaka University, p. 24 (1979)
5.10 G. Brederlow, R. Brodmann, K. Eidmann, H. Krause, M. Nippus, R. Petsch, R. Volk, S. Witkowski, K.J. Witte: Report PLF 5, Projektgruppe für Laserforschung, Garching (1979)
5.11 A.E. Siegman, D.J. Kuizenga, Opto-Electronics 6, 43 (1974)
5.12 M. Nippus: Opt. Commun. 33, 80 (1980)
5.13 H.J. Baker, J.J. Bannister, T.A. King: J. Phys. E. 14, 579 (1981)
5.14 M.M. Howland, S.J. Davis, W.L. Gagnon: Report UCRL-82538, Lawrence Livermo Laboratory (1979)
5.15 G. Mourou, W. Knox: Appl. Phys. Lett. 35, 492 (1979)
5.16 W.W. Simmons, D.R. Speck, J.T. Hunt: Appl. Opt. 17, 999 (1978)
5.17 J.T. Hunt, J.A. Glaze, W.W. Simmons, P.A. Renard: Appl. Opt. 17, 2053 (1978)
5.18 W.H. Lowdermilk, D. Milam: Appl. Phys. Lett. 36, 891 (1980)
5.19 S.P. Mukherjee, W.H. Lowdermilk: Appl. Opt. 21, 293 (1982)
5.20 L.M. Cook, W.H. Lowdermilk, D. Milam, J.E. Swain: Appl. Opt. 21, 1482 (1982)
5.21 K. Eidmann, G. Brederlow, P. Brodmann, R. Sigel, R. Solk, S. Witkowski, K.J. Witte: Report PLF 4, Projektgruppe für Laserforschung, Garching (1978
5.22 V.A. Gaidash, G.A. Kirillow, S.B. Kormer, S.G. Lapin, V.I. Sheminkin, V.K. Shirigin: Zh. Eksp. Teor. Fiz. Lett. 20, 243 (1974)
5.23 E. Fill, K. Hohla: Opt. Commun. 18, 431 (1976)
5.24 J.J. Bannister, H.J. Baker, T.A. King, W.C. McMaught: Phys. Rev. Lett. 44, 1062 (1980)
5.25 Y.A. Eroshenko, G.A. Kirilov, M.R. Modalov, V.I. Shemyakin, V.K. Sharygin: Sov. J. Quantum Electron. 11, 1222 (1981)
5.26 K.H. Drexhage, U.T. Müller-Westerhoff: IEEE J. Quantum Electron. QE-8, 759 (1972)
5.27 U.T. Müller-Westerhoff: Personal Communication, IBM, San José, CA
5.28 S.P. Batashev, M.O. Galpern, V.A. Katulin, O.L. Lebedev, E.A. Luk'yanets, N.G. Mekkhryakova, V.M. Mizin, V. Yu. Nosach, A.L. Petrov, V.A. Petukhov: Kvantovaya Elektron. 6, 2652 (1979)
5.29 D. Beaupère, J.C. Farcy: Opt. Commun. 27, 410 (1978)

5.30 R.W. Eason, R.C. Greenhow, D.M. Goodall, J.F. Holzwarth: Opt. Commun. 32, 113 (1980)
5.31 Annual Report, Projektgruppe für Laserforschung, Garching p. 46 (1979)
5.32 R.J. Keyes: *Optical and Infrared Detectors*, Springer, Berlin (1977).
5.33 H. Ando, H. Kanbe, T. Kimura, T. Yamaoka, T. Kaneda: IEEE J. Quantum Electron QE-14, 804 (1978)
5.34 M. Feng, J.D. Oberstar, T.H. Windhorn, L.W. Cook, G.E. Stillman, B.G. Streetman: Appl. Phys. Lett. 34, 591 (1979)
5.35 W. Schneider, K. Huebner: Phys. Lett. 53A, 87 (1975)
5.36 S.W. Thomas, G.R. Tripp, L.W. Coleman: Adv. Electronics Electron Phys. 40A, 451 (1976)
5.37 S. Ariga, H. Braendlein, P. Sachsenmeier: Report IPP IV/63, Institut für Plasmaphysik, Garching (1974)
5.38 H.J. Baker, T.A. King: Opt. Commun. 18, 286 (1976)
5.39 R.L. Smith, R.J. Phelan jr.: Appl. Opt. 12, 795 (1973)
5.40 G. Beck: Rev. Sci. Instrum. 47, 849 (1976)
5.41 D.J. Bradley, B. Liddy, A.G. Roddie, W. Sibbett, W.E. Sleat: Adv. Electronics Electron Phys. 33B, 1145 (1972)
5,42 M.A. Palmer, R.E. Palmer: unpublished results, Sandia Laboratories, Albuquerque, NM
5.43 W. Friedmann, S. Jackel, W. Seka, J. Zimmermann: SPIE 97, 544 (1976)
5.44 J. van Laar: Acta Electron. 6, 215 (1973)
5.45 S.W. Thomas: Proc. 13th Int. Congress High Speed Photography and Photonics, Tokyo, p. 499 (1978)
5.46 H.J. Baker, J.J. Bannister, T.A. King, E.S. Mukhtar: Appl. Opt. 18, 2136 (1979)
5.47 B.R. Holeman, W.M. Wreathall: J. Phys. D1, 1898 (1971)
5.48 J.C. Farcy, D. Beaupère: Rev. Sci. Instrum. 48, 975 (1977)
5.49 E.W. Selwyn: *Photography in Astronomy*, Eastman Kodak, Rochester, NY (1950) p. 62
5.50 A.G.M. Maaswinkel, K. Eidmann, R. Sigel: Phys. Rev. Lett. 42, 1625 (1979)
5.51 F. Amiranoff, R. Fabbro, E. Fabre, C. Garban, J. Virmont, M. Weinfeld: Phys. Rev. Lett. 43, 522 (1979)
5.52 Laser Programm Annual Report, Lawrence Livermore National Laboratory UCRL 50021-80, pp. 7/3-7/53 (1980)
5.53 Quarterly Report; Laboratory for Laser Energetics, University of Rochester: p. 15 (April-June 1981)
5.54 C.M. Ferrar: Appl. Phys. Lett. 12, 381 (1968)
5.55 R. Volk, K. Hohla: Verh. Dtsch. Phys. Ges. paper Q41, p.130 (1975)
5.56 E.E. Fill: Opt. Commun. 33, 321 (1980)
5.57 Laser Program Annual Report, Lawrence Livermore National Laboratory UCRL 50021-80 (1980) Table 2-66, pp. 2/254-2/284
5.58 R.S. Craxton: Opt. Commun. 34, 674 (1980)
5.59 Cleveland Crystals Inc. Information Sheet (1976)

Chapter 6

6.1 G. Brederlow, K.J. Witte, E. Fill, K. Hohla, R. Volk: IEEE J. Quantum Electron. QE-12, 152 (1976)
6.2 K.J. Witte, G. Brederlow, K. Eidmann, R. Volk, E. Fill, K. Hohla, R. Brodmann: In *High Power Lasers and Applications* ed. by K.L. Kompa, H. Walther, Springer Series in Optical Sciences, Vol. 9, (Springer, Berlin, Heidelberg, New York 1978) pp. 142-147

6.3 G. Brederlow, R. Brodmann, K. Eidmann, H. Krause, M. Nippus, R. Petsch, R. Volk, S. Witkowski, K.J. Witte: Report PLF 5, Projektgruppe für Laserforschung, Garching (1979)
6.4 G. Brederlow, R. Brodmann, K. Eidmann, M. Nippus, R. Petsch, S. Witkowski, R. Volk, K.J. Witte: IEEE J. Quantum Electron. QE-16, 122 (1980)
6.5 A.E. Siegmann, D.J. Kuizenga: Opto-ELectronics 6, 43 (1974)
6.6 T. Uchiyama, K.J. Witte: Report PLF 36, Projektgruppe für Laserforschung, Garching (1979)
6.7 K. Eidmann, G. Brederlow, R. Brodmann, R. Petsch, R. Sigel, G. Tsakiris, R. Volk, S. Witkowski: Report PLF 4, Projektgruppe für Laserforschung, Garching (1978)
6.8 K. Eidmann, G. Brederlow, R. Brodmann, R. Petsch, R. Sigel, G. Tsakiris, R. Volk, S. Witkowski: Report PLF 15, Projektgruppe für Laserforschung, Garching (1979)
6.9 J.T. Hunt, J.A. Glaze, W.W. Simmons, P.A. Renard: Appl. Opt. 17, 2053 (1978)
6.10 E.E. Fill, W. Skrlac, K.J. Witte: Opt. Commun. 37, 123 (1981)

Chapter 7

7.1 K.J. Witte, T. Uchiyama: Report MPQ 46, Max-Planck-Institut für Quantenoptik (1981)
7.2 M.A. Gusino: Opt. Commun. 15, 190 (1975)
7.3 G.A. Fisk, M.A. Gusinov, A.K. Hays, T.D. Padrick, R.E. Palmer, J.K. Rice, M.E. Riley, F.K. Truby: Report SAND 78-1071, SANDIA Laboratories (1978)
7.4 Lawrence Livermore National Laboratory: Laser Program Annual Report, UCRL-50021-78, Vol.3, (1978) p. 9-6
7.5 University of Wisconsin, Dept. Nuclear Eng.: Rep. UWFDM-229, (1977) p.4
7.6 K.J. Witte, P. Burkhard, H.R. Lüthi: Opt. Commun. 28, 202 (1979)
7.7 K. Hohla, K.J. Witte: Report IPP IV/90, Max-Planck-Institut für Plasmaphysik (1976)
7.8 D.J. Bernard, W.E. McDermott, N.R. Pschelkin, R.R. Bousek: Appl. Phys. Lett. 34, 40 (1979)
7.9 G.A. Fisk, T.D. Padrick: Report SAND 78-2306, SANDIA Laboratories (1978)
7.10 G.N. Hays, G.A. Fisk: IEEE J. Quantum Electron. QE-17, 1823 (1981)
7.11 G.E. Busch: IEEE J. Quantum Electron. QE-17, 1128 (1981)

Chapter 8

8.1 G. Brederlow, K.J. Witte: Report PLF 19, Projektgruppe für Laserforschung (1979)

Subject Index

I. I. Sobelman

Atomic Spectra and Radiative Transitions

1979. 21 figures, 46 tables. XII, 306 pages
(Springer Series in Chemical Physics, Volume 1)
ISBN 3-540-09082-7

Contents: Elementary Information on Atomic Spectra: The Hydrogen Spectrum. Systematics of the Spectra of Multielectron Atoms. Spectra of Multielectron Atoms. - Theory of Atomic Spectra: Angular Momenta. Systematics of the Levels of Multielectron Atoms. Hyperfine Structure of Spectral Lines. The Atom in an External Electric Field. The Atom in an External Magnetic Field. Radiative Transitions.-References.- List of Symbols. - Subject Index.

This volume is continued by *Excitation of Atoms and Broadening of Spectral Lines* published as Volume 7 in this series.

"...this book presents a wealth of information about the quantum mechanics of free atoms...it is nearly a must."

Applied Optics

"...is an essential book for any science library and a very valuable text for any specialist in atomic physics..."

Contemporary Physics

I. I. Sobelman, L. A. Vainshtein, E. A. Yukov

Excitation of Atoms and Broadening of Spectral Lines

1981. 34 figures, 40 tables. X, 315 pages
(Springer Series in Chemical Physics, Volume 7)
ISBN 3-540-09890-9

Contents: Elementary Processes Giving Rise to Spectra. — Theory of Atomic Collisions. - Approximate Methods for Calculating Cross Sections.- Collisions Between Heavy Particles. - Some Problems of Excitation Kinetics. - Tables and Formulas for the Estimation of Effective Cross Sections. - Broadening of Spectral Lines.- References.- List of Symbols.- Subject Index. - Errata for volume 1 of this series.

Here is a systematic treatment of the theory of elementary processes, responsible for the excitation of atomic spectra and for spectral line broadening. In dealing with the theory of spectral line broadening, the main emphasis is on problems of contemporary research, such as high-resolution laser spectroscopy, laser frequency and wavelength measurements, plasma physics, and astrophysics.
Atomic excitation processes are investigated comprehensively, presenting efficient and useful methods of approximation for the calculation and estimation of cross-sections. Numerous tables provide the results of calculations for various excitation processes.

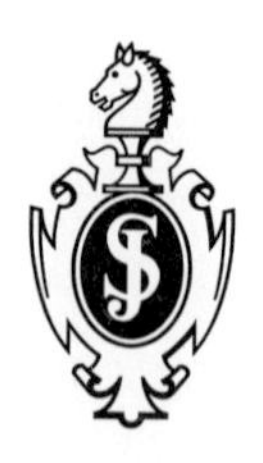

Springer-Verlag
Berlin
Heidelberg
New York